cancer
widow

cancer widow

A nurse practitioner and her husband
navigate the health care system
after his diagnosis of stage four cancer

lynn kelly devlin
with jacquelyn b. fletcher

DEVLIN PUBLISHING
Dover, NH

Disclaimer

This book includes information gathered from many different sources and personal experience. It is published for general reference and not intended to be a substitute for medical advice from your personal health care provider. The book is sold with the understanding that neither the author nor publisher is engaged in rendering any medical, legal, or psychological advice. The publisher and author disclaim any personal liability directly or indirectly for advice or information presented within. Although the author and publisher have prepared this manuscript with utmost care and diligence and have made every effort to ensure the accuracy and completeness of the information contained within, we assume no responsibility for errors, inaccuracies, omissions, or inconsistencies.

© 2012 Lynn Kelly Devlin

All rights reserved. No part of this publication may be reproduced, stored in retrieval system, or transmitted in any form or by any means electronic, mechanical, photocopying, recording or otherwise, without the prior written permission of the publisher.

Published by
Devlin Publishing
P.O. Box 363
Dover, NH 03861
Phone: 603.343.4409
Fax: 603.343.4504

Publisher's Cataloging-in-Publication Data
Devlin, Lynn Kelly.

    Cancer widow : a nurse practitioner and her husband navigate the health care system after his diagnosis of stage four cancer / Lynn Kelly Devlin, with Jacquelyn B. Fletcher. – Dover, NH : Devlin Pub., 2012.

    p. ; cm.

    ISBN13: 978-0-9852873-0-6

    1. Devlin, Kevin. 2. Cancer—Patients—Biography. 3. Medical care—United States. 4. Palliative treatment—United States. 5. Hospice care—United States. 6. Devlin, Lynn Kelly. I. Title. II. Fletcher, Jacquelyn B.

RC265.6.D47 D47 2012
362.1969940092—dc23   2012901955

FIRST EDITION

Project coordination by Jenkins Group, Inc.
www.BookPublishing.com

Production Manager: Leah Nicholson
Creative Director: Yvonne Fetig Roehler
Cover Design: Chris Rhoads
Interior Design: Brooke Camfield
Copyeditor: Tom Wilkens
Lynn Devlin's Author Photo: Ann H. Grinnell
Jacquelyn Fletcher's Author Photo: Joanna Prosser Photography

Printed in the United States of America
16 15 14 13 12 • 5 4 3 2 1

Dedication

To Kevin

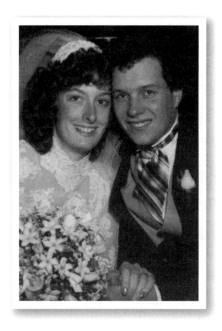

contents

chapter one: widow lady   1
chapter two: missed diagnosis   3
chapter three: holding hands   10
chapter four: to work   19
chapter five: treatment   25
chapter six: who is this man?   36
chapter seven: gradual decline   42
chapter eight: planning a funeral   47
chapter nine: reconnection   51
chapter ten: is this a love story?   57
chapter eleven: the final weekend   62
chapter twelve: saying goodbye   76
chapter thirteen: the soggy year   86
chapter fourteen: alone   93
chapter fifteen: waking up   104
chapter sixteen: just five more minutes   112

about the author   119

CANCER

Cancer is a group of more than one hundred diseases. The definition includes any cluster of abnormal cells growing in your body. Cancer is a stealthy, insidious disease that is often found incidentally—you go in for a mammogram and you come out with news of a suspicious shadow on your x-ray. You go in for a routine colonoscopy and discover you have cancer.

At stage one, there are usually no symptoms. In stage two, cancer is sometimes found while looking for something else. In stage three, people can feel lumps and bumps. They might have funky abdominal pains, coughs, night sweats, or unintentional weight loss.

All of these symptoms are easy to dismiss. "I have a cold or stomach flu," people might think. Unfortunately, we find cancer when it has already reached stage four. By this time, it has often metastasized: moved from its place of origin to other spots throughout the body. That's when people start having symptoms that are hard to ignore, such as pain, a worsening cough, terrible diarrhea, or constipation. Someone might have a nagging backache for months and dismiss it, attributing it to weeding or shoveling too much. If you unintentionally lose more than ten percent of your body weight within a year, then something is going on. Cancer is a wasting disease, and unintentional weight loss is one of its clues.

By the time someone is diagnosed with stage four cancer, there are more than 100,000,000 cancer cells in their body. It's important to know what stage the cancer is in, as it guides the doctors in their choice of treatments.

chapter one
widow lady

We lived in a small town in New Hampshire where my husband, Kevin, knew half the people in town, and I knew everyone else. A few weeks after his death, I stopped at our local grocery store. I didn't need a cart for the few items on my list. I listlessly gathered two bananas, a couple of tomatoes, and some lunchmeat. We had always eaten wheat bread, but that day I wanted something different. On impulse, I grabbed an overpriced loaf of organic wheat berry, olive bread.

While in line at the cash register, I heard a buzzing disturbance behind me. I turned and saw a woman I knew near the end of a long refrigerated case, leaning close to her husband. She pointed at me. "That's her," she said. "That's the widow lady."

I looked down at myself—there were the same khaki pants, cotton shirt, and black flats I usually wore. I was only forty-six years old. Still a mother. Still a nurse. Still me. But with a new identity. *Widow lady*, I whispered to myself.

LOVE

A strong love is not a defense against death.

chapter two

missed diagnosis

"I'm fine. My doctor says I have allergies," Kevin said after seeing his family physician. He'd taken a half day at work and driven straight home after the appointment.

"I'm just going to take a bit of a rest. Come and get me in twenty minutes," he said. He settled on the couch and looked at me. "I'm going to shake this off."

But after resting, he didn't feel refreshed. For more than a year, he'd sporadically woken at night drenched in sweat. For the first time in his life, he shed weight without even trying.

Every day for years, he ate the same sandwich for lunch at a little bakery and sandwich shop across the street from General Electric (GE) where he worked—chicken salad with tomatoes. We would meet there a few times a week to spend a quiet moment together. Suddenly concerned co-workers started buying him lunch, assuming he was working too hard and not eating enough.

Some nights, I woke him out of nightmares. He'd never had bad dreams before, but now he wrestled with unseen monsters. I tried to comfort him.

"It's okay. It was just a dream." I changed the sheets soaked with sweat, and we closed our eyes once more.

This isn't right, I thought. *Something is wrong.*

Until then, the changes had been so subtle that I hadn't noticed them. It was like raising a child. You don't see them gradually growing bigger every day, until one afternoon their pants are several inches too short.

The doctor attributed Kevin's symptoms and thirty-five-pound weight loss to allergies. It was a bad allergy year, with lots of rain, mud, mold, and fungus. Kevin tried a bunch of different over-the-counter allergy medications. They didn't work.

When he developed a horrific sore throat on one side, his doctor tested him for strep throat. The test was negative, but the doctor gave him antibiotics anyway. When nothing happened, they prescribed another antibiotic. When that didn't work, they went back to the first antibiotic and tried it again.

"It's those cats," Kevin said.

We'd recently adopted two cats. Kevin didn't want the pets, but I'd grown up with cats and he agreed to let me have them. I loved the cats. Kevin blamed them for his constant nasal congestion.

I kept setting up appointments with an ear, nose, and throat doctor (ENT), but Kevin cancelled each time, claiming he was too busy to go.

Honey, allergies don't cause weight loss. Why won't you listen to me?

Kevin knew something was dreadfully wrong, but he didn't want to face it.

"I'm just tired from traveling. It was a long flight," he would say, time and again.

You never used to be tired.

When the nosebleeds started, they came suddenly. They'd last for up to thirty minutes and make big clotty messes. The last nosebleed was the worst. It was mid-November, around the time of Kevin's birthday. We were out for supper with some friends: a nurse practitioner friend of mine and her husband. As we talked, I noticed a few drops of blood on Kevin's plate. He hadn't realized his nose was bleeding. I passed him a packet of tissues, but he bled through them all. Then the blood covered his hand. It was everywhere. The bleeding wouldn't stop.

Kevin rushed out of the dining room while I put some ice cubes in a napkin to hold on the bridge of his nose. Once we were outside, Kevin's fear burst through his normal bravado. "What's going on? What's happening?"

"*Please* go to the ENT." I pressed the cold napkin firmly on his nose.

"I will," he finally said.

We returned to the dining room once the nosebleed stopped, but Kevin couldn't eat. The evening was spoiled. We drove home, worried and scared.

After postponing for nearly a year, Kevin finally kept an appointment with the ENT. Kevin sat in a recliner while I perched in a puny little chair next to him. The doctor was very much an old-fashioned physician. He wore a white lab jacket, a tie, and beautifully tailored pants. He was about seventy years old and treated us with paternal superiority, but he was the doctor who spoke the most truth to us.

He strapped the light on his head, like a coal miner's lamp, and looked into Kevin's mouth.

"Oh my God." The doctor stepped back. He checked Kevin's neck and found enlarged lymph nodes.

What? What is it?

"It looks like cancer," he said. We'll need to get a biopsy, blood work, and CAT scans." The doctor went to find his nurse. We followed him out, not speaking, not knowing what to do. Kevin sat down. He shook his head, looking lost and alone. It was Thanksgiving week.

I waited with my daughter, Katie, in the family area. It was a few days into December, and Kevin was preparing to undergo a biopsy in the same-day surgery unit. He acted brave in the prep room. He even agreed to try a Reiki treatment, though he'd never heard of the calming energy work before. It helped relax him, and he started acting loopy and silly. We tried hard to maintain a light-hearted atmosphere for our daughter and for each other.

The anesthesiologist walked in. He was a round man with a shiny face. His blue mask hung down on his chest, the elastic stretched around his neck. He wanted to examine my husband carefully. If Kevin couldn't breathe during the exploratory procedure, they would have to put a ventilator tube down his throat. He asked Kevin to open his mouth.

After examining his throat, the anesthesiologist stood behind my husband. "It's going to be difficult to intubate you during the procedure, but we need an emergency backup plan in case the area collapses during the biopsy."

The smile fell from Kevin's face. Instantly, the room went from surreally cheerful to grim. The anesthesiologist patted Kevin on the shoulder.

"How you go under anesthesia is how you wake up."

Ever the optimist, Kevin tried to shake off his fear.

I should have signed him out right then.

After a short time, the nurse escorted Katie and me to a small waiting room, where we waited for Kevin to wake up. The ear, nose, and throat specialist followed us in his sharply pressed pants and shiny dress shoes. I knew the ENT personally since we were both members of the same medical community.

"I'm sorry to tell you, but it's stage four cancer. He probably won't live six months."

I felt like I was falling to the ground. I could feel the cold slap of tile against my legs. But I didn't fall then. Not on the outside.

Sweet Jesus, not this.

I did the only thing I knew how to do in that moment. Like a good wife and nurse, I shook his hand and thanked him.

His look was cold. "How could this have happened at your house?" he asked. His words felt like slaps.

I froze, thinking, *Stage four . . . stage four . . . is that good or bad?*

The doctor didn't explain the stages of cancer and I didn't ask any questions. I was a nurse, after all. But that day, in that room, I knew no more than anyone else.

I sifted through years of medical training in my mind.

Stage four is as bad as it gets.

It means six months to live or less.

Where the hell were we during stages one, two, and three?

I handed Katie my credit card.

"Go buy your dad a recliner and the biggest TV you can find." I said.

The store delivered and installed them both in our bedroom that same day.

I stared out the window of the cancer center at the snow and the naked, black branches of the trees, gripping the telephone.

"Kevin has cancer," I said. My mother listened on the other end. She was in the men's department of Macy's and had just bought Kevin a Christmas sweater he wouldn't need. I repeated myself, "It's stage four . . . he has stage four cancer . . . it's stage four."

Eventually I hung up, and the tears came. They wouldn't stop. The hospital staff saw me crying on their security cameras and sent a nurse to talk to me. She was my neighbor, Jennifer. I don't remember a word she said, but her presence helped.

Later on, I was glad I cried that day. It was one of my few opportunities to cry while Kevin rode the cancer treatment hamster wheel.

When I finally saw my husband, we clutched each other, sobbing. And then we kissed. Hard. Straight on the lips. Like we did the first time we met.

ADVOCATE

The bitch who holds the hospital door shut so the patient can have some peace.

chapter three
holding hands

I was dating a boy named Bob and attending classes at Northeastern University in Boston. One late September weekend, Bob asked me to return early from a weekend visiting family in Rhode Island. He and a group of his friends were gathering in the revolving bar at the Hyatt Regency hotel in Cambridge. It boasted the best views of the Charles River, downtown Boston, and the brownstones of Cambridge, while the bar slowly revolved 360 degrees. Since it was 1980, I wore a fabulous puffy white disco dress with purple flowers.

The elevator doors opened, and Bob and I took a dizzying step onto the revolving floor. A group of people surged forward to greet us. Bob spotted his dear friend, Linda, standing shoulder-to-shoulder with her boyfriend, Kevin. Bob hugged her and kissed her cheek.

Then Linda introduced us. "Kevin, you know Bob. And this is Lynn."

Kevin.

He was taller than me by only an inch and wore his dark, curly hair cut short.

"If Bob can kiss Linda, then I can kiss Lynn," Kevin said. Before I could react, he pulled me into a tight embrace and kissed me. Hard. Right on the lips. Instantly I felt a visceral, chemical reaction. Something deep inside me said *I recognize you.*

That night he walked me home along the September streets of Boston. The next day he called. After that we were inseparable.

Kevin loved holding hands. He held mine as we took long walks together and explored the city. We used our student discounts to see shows and go for late-night pizza runs. My favorite spot was Brigham's Ice Cream. Time and again, we walked from the Northeastern campus through the Prudential Center to the Christian Science reflecting pool. Once inside the ice cream shop, we ordered a brownie sundae with two spoons. Kevin demonstrated how he thought rich people ate. With his napkin *just so* and his pinky extended, he spooned dainty bits of ice cream into his mouth. I cracked up every time. His sparkling green eyes were so alive with his laughter.

I've known you forever, I thought. I could say anything to him. He could say anything to me. We ate our sweets and dreamed of our future together. Someday we would be those rich people we mocked.

It was the beginning.

We dated for about eighteen months. I was two years younger than Kevin, so he graduated before me from his engineering program. He took a job with GE in their management training program, which meant he'd be reassigned to a different city every two years. His first assignment was in Gahanna, Ohio. He loved it, but missed me. He frequently called and sent cards and letters. We visited each other whenever we could.

Our visits were fantastically romantic. They started with phone calls back and forth while we planned our next exciting adventure. One time, I flew to see him in Columbus, Ohio. I walked off the plane as Kevin waited for me at the end of the gangway. (It was back when you could still pick people up at their arrival gate.) As soon as our eyes locked, his face lit up with the grin I loved so much. I hurried to him and he pulled me close into a tight hug. Then he grabbed my bag, took my hand, and we headed out to experience the city.

Kevin was proud of himself because he had managed to get reservations at one of the fanciest restaurants in town. Meal prices were only listed on the man's copy of the menu. We dressed up. I wore the same flowered dress I'd worn the night we met in Boston. He wore a suit jacket. We felt so grown up on our big-city date.

Are you going to propose? I wondered, as butterflies fluttered in my stomach all night. But he didn't. Not yet.

The next day, we went to an arboretum and walked among the flowers and plants and trees. We knew our time together was ending soon. That evening, Kevin drove me to the airport. We held each other tightly, tears flooding both our faces.

"I love you," he whispered urgently. "I miss you already."

And then I flew back home, wishing the days away so I could see him again.

At Christmas, I was sure he'd propose. He didn't.

But when he flew to Boston for Easter, he had the diamond ring in his pocket. He'd heard somewhere that before you propose, you should prepare to spend four weeks of your salary on the diamond. Kevin always followed the rules, so that's what he did. He saved up four weeks of his salary and bought me the perfect engagement ring.

holding hands

Every time Kevin flew into Boston, I picked him up and we'd spend a day together. Since I hated driving, he'd take the wheel and drive us to my parents' house in Rhode Island. Then we'd drive to Philadelphia to see his family. After that we'd head back to Boston together. We always went to Legal Sea Foods, right on the Boston harbor, for our anniversaries and special occasions. On our Easter visit in 1982, we headed to our usual spot: a U-shaped banquette with a view of the aquarium. I ordered scrod and Kevin got the clam chowder. After dinner, we chose a chocolate-covered ice cream dessert. Once our decadent treat arrived, Kevin took out the ring.

"Today is April ninth. Will you marry me on October ninth?"

"I would be honored," I said, grinning. We kissed, and everyone in the restaurant cheered.

We married on October 9, 1982. I became Kevin's wife, in health and in sickness until death parted us.

The early years were the sweetest. Kevin's career was on the upswing. He put me through school so I could finish my nursing degree. We were transferred to a different state every two years—New York, Pennsylvania, and New Hampshire. Discovering each new place and making it our home, became an adventure that connected us. Each time, we had to reestablish who we were, and we loved it. It was just the two of us together, exploring the world.

We'd find the coffee shops, test the restaurants, and meet new people. As we got to know a city, we avoided the big chains. Instead we'd look for small, family-owned places where we could chat with the owners. And in every city, we made a point of finding a hot spot with a tasty happy hour, so we wouldn't have to make supper.

We were both close with our families, and every Sunday we'd each call home to talk to our parents and siblings. Both of us wanted children. We had our first daughter when I was twenty-six and Kevin was twenty-eight.

After Katie was born, we continued to go on our long walks. We lived in an apartment, and Kevin would bundle the baby up in her carriage and carefully carry the entire thing down the steps, every inch the doting dad.

As I watched them together, my heart filled. *I love my life.*

Our second daughter came four years later, and she was just as precious to us. We'd promised each other that when we started a family, we'd settle down somewhere and stop moving around. After our first daughter was born, we moved two more times before we found a place we thought we could call home for long enough to raise our children. The small town in New Hampshire seemed well established. The brick buildings and old-world history felt grounded and solid. A beautiful river ran through the middle of downtown.

Besides beauty, the town offered everything I thought we needed to raise a family. There were great swimming pools, dance and gym classes, and fun opportunities to integrate with the community. We wanted a church we could raise our kids in and a town large enough to support our careers. Ultimately, we wanted to become locals and that's exactly what we did. We bought a starter home, and suddenly our entire lives fit within a ten-mile loop.

In 1996, we moved into Kevin's dream house. It was a colonial-style executive home with blue siding, white window trim, and a bright red door. The pie-shaped property was once an apple orchard, and Kevin planted several trees, a lilac, and a row of evergreens. He planted and lovingly tended an antique pear tree. The town was safe. The kids ran free and played with the dog. We threw block parties at the end of the street in the cul-de-sac with all the neighbors.

During summer months, Kevin and I attended concerts in the downtown band shell every Friday. In the winter, Kevin powered up his beloved snow blower. He cleared our driveway, the fire hydrant, and the neighbors' driveways. He loved it. It was picture perfect—for a while.

Then came the busy time: the time in our marriage when things became difficult. When we argued over parenting differences. When we kept saying to each other, "We'll have more time for each other later." We kept up our date nights, but something always came before our marriage.

Kevin started to feel pressure at work. Because of the family, he turned down jobs in Puerto Rico and Brazil and once you decline a promotion, they start to pass you over. Still, he had to keep traveling, so the girls and I grew accustomed to his absence. Every three months, he left for two to three weeks. He took frequent overnight trips and sometimes traveled to Mexico for weeks at a time. He called us every night, but when he returned home there was definitely an adjustment period.

Eventually, we settled into a pattern that felt unbreakable. Kevin wanted to have a say in things at home, but felt like he intruded on the routines I'd set up for me and the girls while he was gone. We were set in our rhythm—driving to dance classes, girl scouts, Sunday school—but Kevin was out of step. He often felt like a guest when he returned, so he wasn't pleasant to be around. I'm sure I was snotty to him when I insisted on the routine I'd established. I remember saying, "Let's be done. We can separate. No harm. No foul." But as soon as we'd say things like that to each other, we'd both make an effort and our marriage would get better for a while . . . until it fell apart again.

During the last five years of our marriage, there were many times I didn't mind him leaving on another business trip.

You used to have so much energy. What is happening to you? You used to be so fun. I thought he was going through a mid-life crisis.

Kevin's dream house sat on an acre of beautiful land. Since he had grown up in Philadelphia without a lawn, he worked on our yard as often as possible. Every night he came home, ate supper, and walked the perimeter of our property. When we first moved there, I would walk with him, but I stopped after our relationship became strained.

The last year of his life, he asked me to walk with him again, and I begrudgingly tagged along. Each time he showed me what he planted.

That antique pear tree is more precious to you than me, I thought one night.

I didn't know he was marking his time. Perhaps he didn't either, but I think he knew he was in trouble. His energy wasn't the same. He'd stopped doing the things he loved. I kept pushing him.

"Why don't you go outside to weed or plant something?"

"No. I'm going to go rest for a bit."

I thought maybe he was depressed. Now, though, I know he'd had the cancer for four to six years before we found out. So when he kept refusing to do things he loved, it was the cancer thickening his blood, toying with his metabolism, making him too tired to get out of his chair.

Touching was always part of our marriage, even during the rough patches. Kevin would think I was mad at him if we didn't have physical contact or sit close to each other on the couch. We had turned into one person, one unit. But in the last year, when Kevin was feeling so lousy, our sex life all but disappeared.

On October 9, 2006, our twenty-fourth wedding anniversary, Kevin unloaded the dishwasher. After he put away the plates and glasses, he looked at me and flashed a knowing grin with his fabulous smile. Instantly, we tapped back into our old selves, as if the last few years had never happened.

I know this version of you. I like this version. I know what you want. I grinned back.

INFORMED CONSENT

Before you begin any kind of cancer treatment, you must read the documents that explain the possible effects of drugs and radiation. Anything you do risks bad consequences. If you accept treatment, make sure you know the intent or goal of the treatment. Is it intended to cure, or is it to relieve symptoms?

You can read about these horrible things, but you never think they will happen to you. You think if you just go along with the rules and do everything right, you'll beat the cancer. You think the risk of treatment is a small price to pay for extending your life, so you sign the document and accept the risk. But if that extra time is poor quality time, is it worth it?

chapter four
to work

"I'm an engineer," Kevin said shortly after his diagnosis. "I don't really understand this medical thing. You handle that. I look at cancer as nothing more than a production problem, and I can fix a production problem."

He dismissed me that day from being his wife. So I suppressed the wifely part of me—the terrified part—and went to work as the nurse.

When I was born, my great-grandmother said to my mother, "She looks like a nurse." When I was three, I told my mother I was going to be a nurse. Each Halloween I dressed as a nurse. I never wanted to be anything else. I volunteered in high school as a candy striper the second I could. Later in my teens, I worked at a hospice, and after that a mental illness facility. Eventually I became a family nurse practitioner, sometimes working with cancer patients. Due to the fragmentation of care within the health care system, I saw cancer patients for other things, such as diabetes, bronchitis, or sore throats.

I had experience. This is why that well-dressed doctor asked me the same question I've asked myself a million times since: *How could this have happened at my house?*

> I am a palliative care nurse practitioner. This appointment has been scheduled because you're having a very bad day. If you're lucky, you'll be well enough to participate meaningfully in this meeting. If not, then you're lying in a hospital bed, probably tethered to several noisy machines. Plastic tubes are stuffed in every orifice we can access. If they've been accessed too many times before and are worn out, then we will drill into your body, with imprecise tools, until we find a pipeline. We will drop IV fluids into your arm, drip baby formula down your nose, and insert a catheter to drain your urine. Don't even ask me what happens when you have a bowel movement.
>
> "This meeting has been scheduled . . ." I open every meeting the same way. It gives me a couple of minutes to assess the people sitting in the room. Everyone at the family meeting is tense. They've been waiting a while. Nothing in a hospital happens on schedule. Patients get upset about this. Silly patients. There are more important things to worry about.
>
> "Your referral was faxed over this morning. I've had the opportunity to review your chart," I say. What I mean is: I've reviewed your *entire* chart, which is probably inches thick with X-rays, CAT scans,

MRIs, and blood work results from the last few years of your life. I will, most likely, be the only person who has ever looked at your entire chart. The communication between people in different medical specialties is notoriously poor. But you may already have a sense of that.

The family huddles around the bed. Sometimes the patient and his wife hold hands. I like that. Showing affection indicates strength. It shows a tight bond. I think these two will speak in a shared voice.

I take the only available seat, strategically placed by the head of the bed, so we can hear clearly and look directly at each other. Open, direct communication is best. Now it's time to hear your personal story.

"I've spent the better part of the morning reviewing your chart," I say. I wave my handwritten notes. "I know what I want to say, but first I want to make sure you all know why we're here."

The family exhales collectively. Folks sit back a little in their chairs, adjust their clothing, and settle in. I am not the grim reaper they were expecting.

I am very tall. I was thin for my height when I was younger, but pregnancy forever changed that. Now I'm proportional. I love beautiful clothes with classic lines and soft fabric. I almost always wear a skirt or dress. At work, a crisp, tailored lab coat acts as a protective layer between me and my patients.

I can feel my personality pull back. As each button of my lab coat is fastened, I become a bit more reserved. I am not here to make friends. By the end of my workday, I will have created a wake of upset. No one wants to be here.

My job is to shed light on your clinical scenario. I help you pull together all the information you're getting so that you can understand it. I also discuss what the trajectory of your disease looks like. I have ninety minutes to do it. But you won't know that.

"What do you want to know?" you ask me.

"I already know you haven't felt well for the better part of a year. Tell me what you understand about your physical condition."

I invite you to dismiss anyone from the meeting who you don't want to share everything about everything with, but you won't want anyone to leave.

I know what your chart says, but I don't know you. Your family members may pipe up, but I will shush them. Now it is your turn to speak. You tell me what it's like for you day-to-day. Are you able to walk independently? If so, how far? What are you able to eat? No, not last week, today. Can you groom yourself? Are you doing any chores? I can see by your daughter's reaction that she didn't know you needed help in the shower, or that you are no longer driving because you feel too weak.

Stop the meeting. Where are the tissues? We take a break, which throws the meeting off for a while. When the family regains their composure, we continue.

You tell me you love your work, you love your family. You will fight this cancer with everything you've got. I confirm that the medical establishment will help you do just that. The rest of the family cheers Dad's bravery. You GO Dad! We are all so proud of you.

I fight the urge to vomit.

STRENGTH

All through Kevin's illness and afterward, I received hundreds of cards from friends, family, and colleagues. The message on one Papyrus card said it all. "Strength: To hold it together when everyone else would understand if you fell apart."

TUMOR BOARD

After a tumor is identified, the doctor surgically removes a piece and sends it to a pathology lab. A technician examines the sample under a microscope. Then the patient's chart and the tumor information go to a tumor board: a group of medical professionals who decide the best treatment option. There are no identifying details on the chart about the patient's identity, just the facts about his body and his cancer. Tumor boards ask questions such as "Are the patient's kidneys and liver okay?" Many different kinds of chemotherapies eat the liver and kidneys faster than the cancer can take them.

Once the tumor board gives its recommendation, the oncologist will carefully explain to the patient what they have, where the tumor is, the extent of their disease, and their treatment options. The patient is presented with several choices. If surgery is an option, that usually is done first. You want to remove the bulk of the cancer. Breast, uterine, and prostate cancer can be cut out. But other cancers, such as leukemia or multiple myloma, are deep in the bone and are only affected by moderating agents. Moderating agents are palliative treatments used to keep the cancer at bay.

Depending on the goal of the treatment, the patient will be offered chemotherapy, the use of drugs to try to beat back the cancer, and radiation therapy, which uses ionizing radiation to damage the DNA of cancer cells. Since most chemotherapy—and all radiation treatment—cannot target cancer cells in particular, they kill healthy cells, too.

chapter five

treatment

And so it started. Our lives evaporated instantly into a round of appointments, sometimes several a day. We met with our local oncologist, who gave Kevin CAT scans, barium swallows, and PET scans. CAT scans are fancy x-rays that show two-dimensional pictures of the inside of our bodies. A barium swallow is a test that includes swallowing barium sulfite, which coats the hollow esophagus so the doctor can examine the upper gastrointestinal tract. PET scans are machines that create three-dimensional images of our insides that show how our body systems are functioning.

After seeing the results of the three tests, the doctor reported grim news. Because of the location of Kevin's cancer in his throat and how advanced it was, he didn't believe that the chemotherapy and radiation he could offer would help. He sent us to Boston, over an hour away, to meet with another cancer specialist at the Dana-Farber Cancer Institute, one of the most famous and well-respected cancer centers in the country.

Boston time is different than local time. A twenty-minute appointment could easily take up to six hours. The CAT scan machines were full, so they sent us to a same-day scanning facility. But the doctors didn't speak English. They spoke in medicalese—and though they were truthful, no matter how carefully I listened, I couldn't understand everything they said.

There were rules to the medical appointments. We were so stressed out and tired. Neither Kevin nor I remembered what the doctor said correctly, so we would argue about what we thought we heard. The brain only absorbs less than fifty percent of what you hear during an office visit (according to the 2008 study "Does Age Really Matter? Recall of Information Presented to Newly Referred Patients With Cancer" in the *Journal of Clinical Oncology*). Because of this, our friend Tina helped out and traveled with us on our trips to Boston. She mediated from the back seat and checked her notes to see exactly what the doctor had said when the visit was over.

First Kevin met with the nurse. Then the social worker. He answered the same questions over and over. "How are you feeling? Have you lost weight? Are you eating?" By the time we finally saw the doctor, we were both exhausted.

Kevin endured another round of tests. The doctor, a dignified man wearing a button-down shirt and a lab coat, offered his treatment options.

"You can do aggressive chemotherapy and radiation. It won't cure you, but it might keep the tumor at bay a little longer. If you decide to do the standard chemo and radiation protocols, you'll be taken within an inch of your life. Or . . ."

I leaned forward in my seat, hoping he would give us the silver bullet I was looking for.

"I'm doing a clinical trial you could join."

Yes! A clinical trial!

We agreed to look at the materials, and the doctor went on his way. The clinical nurse specialist took up the rest of our time explaining the treatment. We went home and reviewed the inches-thick set of documents the nurse had given us on our way out. Kevin could try a new drug that appeared to eat tumors in laboratory mice. The only problem was—it could also eat holes in Kevin's face. No one else had signed up to participate in the trial.

I called the nurse back. "How is this clinical trial going to help Kevin?"

"It's not," the nurse said. "But it could help other people after him."

This was our silver bullet? This?

What I didn't understand was that clinical trials are not only for lucky people. Everyone who has stage four cancer, with very little hope for recovery, is allowed to take part if researchers are studying that kind of cancer.

Since Kevin didn't much care for Swiss cheese, we opted out of the clinical trial. The Boston doctor told us we could do the chemotherapy and radiation in our home town. And that was the last we saw of him.

Chemotherapy is so toxic that a normal IV can't be used because the chemicals will destroy the smaller veins. Because patients will receive chemo so many times, a port is implanted in their body. That way, patients don't have to endure endless needles pricking their skin. The doctor drills into the chest to reach a bigger, thicker-walled vein that handles the drugs better, keeping the patient more comfortable. The port is placed beneath the skin just under the collarbone, with a catheter that connects directly to the vein providing the medical staff instant access for drugs and fluids.

Kevin was signed up for a gastrointestinal (GI) feeding tube next. The doctors had told him that eventually he wouldn't be able to swallow. They had to operate fast because Kevin's immunity would soon be in the tank. Nobody ever talked to us about alternatives to the feeding tube. Usually you are not meant to use a feeding tube indefinitely. The tube was only supposed to be used until Kevin could swallow again—if he could swallow again.

He was in the hospital for five days, waiting for the surgery to insert the tube into his stomach, but the doctors kept putting it off since his lab work was so bad. He didn't have the strength to go through surgery, and he couldn't eat. Finally, the doctor okayed the procedure. My friend Cathy visited us at the hospital.

"What can I do for you?" she asked.

"Nothing, thank you. We're all set," I said, holding tight to Kevin's hand. I'd known Cathy for a long time, though, and she saw a panicked mask on my face. She told me later that, though we faked bravery, I looked petrified and she could see Kevin's pain in his smile. His physical appearance shocked her. His body was so wasted and his skin color had changed.

Cathy left us, but couldn't leave the parking lot. She sat in her car and prayed and cried. She saw a deflated Kevin who she barely recognized, even though she'd seen him only ten days before.

Instead of returning to work, Cathy called to take off a couple of hours. She stopped at a sandwich shop and gathered up food, then returned to the hospital. Kevin had just come back from having the feeding tube put in and I stood out in the hallway. All of a sudden, I saw Cathy walking toward me with a three-inch tall sandwich.

It probably weighed a pound, packed with meat and vegetables. She also brought a bag of chips and a cookie. I ate all of it. I wouldn't have eaten that day if she hadn't fed me.

Kevin wanted to start the chemotherapy right away. He thought that if he cooperated, he'd be cured. In my notes from that time, I wrote: "Chemo will begin on Tuesday, December 26, with an overnight for observation. Thank God! Thank God! Thank God!"

From that day until the very end of his life, Kevin went in for chemotherapy or radiation therapy five days a week, every week. In the waiting room of the cancer center, there was always a woman in a turban. It was probably a different woman every time.

On our first visit, I didn't know waiting room etiquette. When approached by someone while walking down the hall, do I make eye contact or not? Do I give a quick nod or a chipper "good morning?"

Since I'm a nurse, I decided to look people in the eye and smile, but I never asked them how they felt. Wrong question. Sometimes I couldn't tell the patients from the caregivers because everyone in the room had a horrific look in their eyes.

On Kevin's first day of chemotherapy, we checked in to the cancer center. The registration person had no information in Kevin's chart. Nothing since December 7—twenty-one days ago—and she was surprised that Kevin arrived ready to be admitted. We waited for the doctor in the exam room for an hour, overhearing him talk to a nearby patient.

Hurry up and wait.

Then we sat in the waiting room some more, where we discovered that cancer smells. In the cancer center, the smell alone could kill you. The sense of desperation was palpable. I learned that if I had to go to the bathroom, I had to do it early in the day before the vomiting and diarrhea began. The bathrooms were OSHA hazards with brown bits, mucus strands, and wet stains on the toilet seat. Paper towels spilled over the edge of the trash baskets to the floor. As the day progressed, patients vomited in the waiting room. The retching and groans and soft sobbing made the room sound like the fourth ring of Hell.

The distressed patients cleaned up after themselves the best they could, generously spraying the bathroom with a sickly-sweet orange-scented freshener that only made the odor worse. The sick person then had to walk out to face the rest of the waiting patients.

Finally, the nurse led us down a long corridor. It looked like a spa, but instead of massage tables, there were gurneys and geri chairs: reclining, plastic-lined chairs that people could put their feet up in. The newcomers sat in the middle, where everyone could see them hooked up to IVs with the puke buckets in easy reach.

Kevin, and everyone else receiving treatment, took Benedryl before therapy. One day, when we were still new to chemo and sitting in the horrible seats in the middle of the room, I rummaged through my bag filled with a protein drink, bills to pay, and work to do. I realized there was an absence of noise. It was absolutely silent. When I looked around, I saw I was the only one awake.

I was outraged. *Do they all need this much medication? Do they all need to sleep through this?*

It was the same every time.

Just after one of Kevin's chemotherapy appointments, my husband lay in a hospital bed. I sat next to him on the mattress, holding his hand. He'd placed the newspaper I'd brought on his lap and pointed out something funny. We laughed and looked into each other's eyes. Kevin still had his full head of gorgeous brown curls shot through with gray streaks. The chemo had not yet ravaged his body and mind. I didn't hear the doctor's footsteps. All I heard was my husband's warm laughter. But suddenly, the cancer specialist was there, a vaguely irritated look on his face.

Kevin refused to let go of me, pulling me closer still.

"This doesn't look good," the doctor said. He gave us more bad news. Kevin's blood report showed he wasn't healthy enough to go home. He'd have to stay in the hospital. That was the last real laugh we shared.

After our second visit to Dana-Farber, they told us to stop holding hands. They told me to sleep in another bed because the chemo was leaking through Kevin's pores. We had to triple-flush the toilet after he visited the bathroom and wash his laundry in a separate load with a double rinse. No more hugging. No more physical intimacy.

When we were alone, we reassured each other. "It's okay. We've postponed our private time before." And we had. We'd said there'd be more time for us when the kids weren't babies, when the kids were out of preschool, when they weren't in so many lessons, when they passed through adolescence, when we weren't too tired or stressed or pissed off at each other.

We will be physical again when this is over. When I can kiss your lips and not have to brush away the taste of chemo off mine.

We couldn't even hold hands. When I rested mine on the armrest in the car, Kevin could no longer reach his familiar hand out to give me a quick squeeze. We were always good hand holders, and a soft squeeze could mean "I'm sorry," "I love you," or "Let's hurry upstairs." When we held hands, our connection excluded everyone else.

It's just me and you.

Our bond was strong, and it endured the normal moments of disconnection that happen in long marriages. That was part of the reason why coming home to see Kevin with his head shaved was so upsetting to me.

Gone were the swirling, glorious dark curls I had run my hands through so often. Instead, Kevin now sported the close-cropped stubble of a shaved head. His parents and brother came to visit, and they thought they could spare me some pain if they shaved Kevin's head instead. Kevin's brother felt honored to do it. He ran to the local pharmacy and picked up a kit that would get the job done.

Cancer specialists always recommend that you shave your own head because it can give you a sense of a control in an uncontrollable situation. Kevin shaved his head on his own terms, and he actually liked the new look. He'd already collected mounds of hair each morning from his pillow and the shower drain. I understood why he did it. But coming home to this dramatic physical change was a devastating emotional blow for me.

Who is this man? I thought when I first saw him. The shock was intense. I barely recognized the person I'd stood beside for nearly a quarter of a century.

Each time we had an appointment, the oncologist said the same thing after he breezed in with his super tan and wide grin. "How are you doing? You look so good!"

He shook Kevin's hand like a used car salesman.

In my mind I screamed, *Look a little closer! Can't you see he's lost weight? His color is terrible. He can't feel his feet. Listen to his voice. He's got a hot potato voice that sounds like he's juggling one in his throat. It's not the sexy kind of husky voice, it's terrible. LOOK at him!*

The doctor's overly upbeat attitude discouraged Kevin from answering his questions honestly. If the doctor was still smiling after the work he did all day, then Kevin must smile, too. Kevin said he felt better than he really did and kept silent about the symptoms he suffered.

The doctor was a fine man, no doubt, but he wouldn't even sit down. I learned it's a bad sign when they sit down. It's a strategy they teach in medical school: don't sit down or your visit time will go up.

CARE FOR THE CAREGIVER

When my friend Cathy visited Kevin and me in the hospital for his feeding tube insertion, she felt helpless. But in the simple act of picking up a giant sandwich, chips, and a cookie, she gave me such a wonderful gift. Friends often don't know how to lend support during traumatic events. And I couldn't ask for help because I didn't know what I needed.

Cathy saw the panic on my face and knew she couldn't leave without doing something. Making sure I was fed was a clear action she could take. Cathy was so happy she returned to the hospital that day. I was struck by her thoughtfulness. Those few minutes with her while I ate that meal were a few minutes of a different reality.

So many people assume that the caregiver is also caring for herself. The truth is that self-neglect is easy when you're afraid for someone you love.

CHEMOTHERAPY

Chemotherapy is a cocktail of poisonous drugs used to target and kill cancer cells. The cocktail prescribed depends on the kind of cancer and how advanced it is. Though there are some new therapies that target only the cancer cells, most of them are not that sophisticated. Chemotherapists walk a fine line because the drugs hit fast-dividing cells in the body, but they don't discriminate other than that so they hit the healthy cells, too. Administer too much chemotherapy, and you'll kill the patient.

The doctor will prescribe a cocktail of drugs, the strongest ones first, for a certain amount of time. That's called a protocol. If the first protocol doesn't work, they switch to a new cocktail of drugs for a while. That's the second protocol. With each protocol, the chances of the treatment working go down. Typically, there is not a great response to chemotherapy in advanced cancer.

The side effects of chemotherapy are brutal, like some kind of old-fashioned torture. The patient is often nauseated and fatigued. Chemo alters taste buds, so patients can't taste things like they could before the treatment. Chemo eats at nerve endings, so patients often can't feel their hands or feet. And because it aims at rapidly dividing cells, it hits hair follicles, the tongue, and stomach lining.

Salvage chemotherapy is an extremely aggressive form of treatment. Doctors administer high doses of chemo in a massive attack to try to beat the cancer into remission. This is brutal on the patient. It is usually reserved for people who have not responded to treatment or have had a recurrence of cancer. It is also sometimes used in younger patients. This is the form of chemotherapy that Kevin endured.

chapter six

who is this man?

Dealing with a guy who has cancer is hard. The treatment quickly started taking its toll. Kevin felt bad, so he became cranky and irritable. Not normally an anxious guy, he now became overwhelmed if someone gave him too much information. He no longer seemed interested in the kids' stories, concerns, or grades. The problems in our marriage seemed magnified by one thousand percent.

Even though I picked up on a lab error, Kevin thanked me by yelling at me. After waiting for hours while he had yet another CAT scan, he said nothing but caustic comments.

"You're telling the doctors what to do!" he screamed at me late one night. "You pressured the doctor to order the chest scan."

Inside, my resentment and hurt spiraled out of control. *He asked me to do this! But he has no respect for my knowledge. He acts like I'm stupid. From now on, Kevin can handle his illness by himself. If he wants my opinion he can ask. All my questions are answered. He doesn't even know what to ask.*

From now on, there will be no advice, no pressure to go to the emergency room or get hard copies of the lab results or discuss test findings.

Nothing is right for him—the recliner, CAT scans, how much information I share with people. Enough already. Let his family come help.

As he had more exposure to the chemotherapy, his personality changed dramatically. His body became hypersensitive. If I helped him button his nightshirt on, it was never right. The clothing would hurt him, and he'd snap at me.

I realized I couldn't expect Kevin to be the same old person he'd been even a couple of weeks before. The Kevin I knew was disappearing.

I want the old Kevin back, the one who helped out in all the unseen ways that spouses do. The one who showed concern for the kids and me. The one who had an opinion about everything and wasn't afraid to share it and defend it to the floor. I want my husband back.

I couldn't let my guard down. Not for a minute. While I readied myself for the next bad thing to happen, I acted as a buffer for the kids. We were always very open at our house, and if Kevin had a bad lab result, everybody knew. His lab results were never good.

I often think about the kids during that time. I used to skip up our wooden stairs, but when I came home from the hospital, I slowly dragged up them, one foot in front of the other, on my way to tell them more bad news.

Are you mad at me for telling the truth? I wondered. *Do you hate me for always delivering bad news?*

My daughters still needed me. Katie was nineteen and off at college, but home often for visits. Christine was fifteen, a busy high-school student. They both still needed an active parent. They had real needs every day. I knew they wanted normal lives, but they also had to know what was going on.

There was no room for my feelings. No comfort. No way to find a moment of release. So I held on to the stress.

At some point, I started using my therapeutic voice with Kevin. The one I used at work with ill patients. I became very matter-of-fact, sometimes treating him like a child.

I drove on autopilot to the cancer center. The schedule became something to hang on to. I made sure he was on time. Kevin's anxiety hit the roof if we were late. Before Kevin's illness, wherever we went, we would park far away from the door and walk together. At the beginning of the treatment, I parked at the end of the parking ramp, but not very long into it, I made up excuses to drive him up to the front door of the brick building.

"There's no parking. I have to drop you off," I said. He argued at first, saying he was strong enough to walk. But soon, I didn't have to make up a story. The cancer made him so weak. He actually looked pretty good for a while—the treatment gave him ruddy cheeks. But I could see the weakness overtaking him.

The tube feedings were the worst part for both of us. The nurses showed him how to push the sticky, sweet, foul-smelling formula through the tube and directly into his stomach. But he wanted me to do it because it made him nauseated. I agreed. While I pushed the sludge into the tube, I kept my eyes focused on what I was doing while a mantra played in my mind: *Don't look at me. Just keep your eyes closed.*

Kevin's stomach cramped from the formula, so I had to ease it in slowly. He often burped up the smell and taste of the disgusting stuff, and he dreaded those moments. Each feeding tube session took an hour to do. They happened six times a day, every day, on exactly the same schedule.

Sometimes he hiccupped or coughed after I fed him. When he was coughing, he probably aspirated, which means that his saliva got into his lungs and caused him pain. I always felt like I hurt him more than I helped.

Kevin felt so vulnerable and afraid during the tube feedings that he would get upset. I said all the right things: "You're going to be all right." He wasn't all right. I learned to do things quickly and silently. There were days I knew why he kept watching television and refused to look at me. If he looked, we'd both start crying. In those moments, we both knew he wasn't going to get better. We had so much to lose.

CHEMO BRAIN

At first, I was puzzled by Kevin's behavioral changes. We were so deep in the trenches that I didn't realize he was starting to get chemo brain. We'd certainly had arguments in our marriage, like all couples, but this was different. His irritability, forgetfulness, and irrational behavior were our new baseline. I felt hurt and angry when he acted terribly toward me or the kids. I didn't understand that it was the chemo brain making him act like a jerk.

Chemotherapy can trigger the nausea and anxiety centers of your brain. People going through chemotherapy often undergo a personality change. Chemo is like a stick of dynamite. It hits everything. It's not targeted. It hits the good cells and the bad cells. If I'd known that the chemo brain had settled in, I would have been nicer to Kevin, but my feelings were so hurt.

CURE AND SURVIVAL RATES

With advanced stage four cancer, the survival rates are measured for certain time periods, usually between two and five years. According to Paul Glare and Nicholas A. Christakis, the editors of *Prognosis in Advanced Cancer* (Oxford University Press), the majority of people with advanced cancer do not live past two years.

If this book were about earlier stages of cancer, we'd be having a different conversation. In the earlier stages, cure is the goal, followed by surveillance for recurrence of the disease. That conversation is about how you make living with cancer part of your everyday life.

Estimating the remaining length of someone's life is called prognostication. Many doctors are uncomfortable telling a family how long their loved one has to live, but prognostication is an evidence-based science.

We would have loved the opportunity to talk with a palliative care expert. If someone would have given us Kevin's prognosis, including the expected trajectory of his disease, we could have chosen between aggressive medical intervention or quality of life.

The ENT doctor was the only person who ever warned us that Kevin's time was short. Now I know that Kevin had a ninety-nine percent chance of dying within two years of his diagnosis. I wish I'd known that then. The treatment would have been different, less intense. No salvage chemotherapy.

chapter seven
gradual decline

I don't remember exactly when we stopped laughing. But from the moment Kevin was diagnosed to the day he died in March, I don't remember laughing much. Still, life had to go on at home. One of my girls directed a play at school. The other learned how to skate. But my mind was so preoccupied that I missed these things. I didn't celebrate with them. Our house used to be where the girls' friends came after school. It was a happy, busy place. All that stopped once we found out Kevin was sick.

The way we lived radically changed within just a month of the diagnosis. I used to cook every night, and I enjoyed cooking for the people I loved. But Kevin became so sick from the treatment that he couldn't take the smell of food. Instead, I gave the kids money and told them to go out for pizza but to not bring the food home. For dinner, I ate a bowl of Cheerios and a vitamin pill. The disease distorted our lives so deeply that when Kevin was hospitalized for dehydration, we actually felt relief. We could eat in our house. We could make noise. I could sleep again.

After school, Christine took the bus to the hospital whenever Kevin was admitted. She walked into the hospital room as if it were completely normal. She'd throw her bag down, and we'd walk to the cafeteria to eat so at least I knew she'd eaten something nutritious that day. I watched the childhood slip out of her once her daddy got sick. This was our new normal. We acclimated to the hospital schedule. If it was Tuesday, we knew it was beef stew night. Desserts we saved and ate when we got home. We stayed until visiting hours were over. At 8:00 p.m., we ate our treats in front of the television to decompress.

Around the holidays, Kevin rallied. "Let's keep things as normal as we can," he said. The holidays had always been a time of wonderful togetherness for our entire family. For many years, we had dinner and took Christmas photos at Wentworth By The Sea, a nearby hotel built in 1874 that overlooked the Atlantic Ocean.

We knew we couldn't do that this year, but I invited friends over and cooked my famous prime rib roast. It was Kevin's favorite recipe, the one meal he always wanted on special occasions. During the evening, my girlfriends took turns slipping upstairs to see Kevin for a bit, while the kids stayed downstairs with my family and me.

One of my friends rushed down the stairs.

"Kevin vomited," she said.

I ran to our bedroom and helped clean him up. He was sick from the smell of the dinner. Kevin didn't have to ask me not to cook prime rib again.

I was surprised he never asked me, "Did you get the oil changed?" On Saturdays, he always cleaned both cars and drove them each to the little gas station in town, where he filled them with gas and checked the oil. After he got sick, none of those old chores were on his radar anymore. He really checked out the day he was diagnosed. He turned inward, carefully guarding his thoughts and emotions.

We never had any conversations about the kids. He knew I would take good care of them. Kevin always loved the girls so much, and they were all close. The three of them loved sports and always went to hockey and football games together. But his last conversations with his daughters were difficult. He was irritable with both of them. He groused at one for leaving the computer on and complained to the other about how he felt ignored when she called home. At times, I felt the girls were held hostage. Though the house was their home, too, they couldn't cook, couldn't make noise, couldn't have their own concerns or upsets.

I didn't see it at the time, but as Kevin deteriorated, I began caring for more and more of his needs.

"Could you help me put on my sneakers? Could you tie them? Could you help with my socks?" he'd ask, because he couldn't feel his fingers. No one thing happened that triggered me to think we were on a slippery slope of his gradual decline. I didn't see that it was taking both of us to live his life. I dressed him, fed him, and brought him everything he needed.

There was no time to just be a kid in all of that.

Kevin was so kind to the girls their entire lives, and he would have hated it if all they remembered were the last few weeks. In a way, though, if they hadn't had those last stressful words, it might have been harder on the kids. And Kevin. He displayed a common type of behavior called nest spoiling. I found it easier to think of Kevin as a jerk then, but he wasn't a jerk at heart. I think his crankiness and disconnection with the kids helped him leave them. And me.

I suppose that cooking a prime rib around someone undergoing chemotherapy wasn't the best idea, but I hadn't grasped the reality or gravity of my new situation. Kevin spent more and more time in the hospital, yet nobody explained to us that this was a bad sign. My job was to run back and forth to the hospital, clean up puke, stay out of the line of fire, and try to keep things normal. But things were not normal. The disease progressed.

You can only have a CAT scan every few months to check the progression of the cancer. Kevin was sick from the chemo and sick from the disease, but we accepted it as the new—temporary—normal. Kevin was willing to suffer the side effects in the hope that he was in the one percent that survived.

In my head, the treatment was only going to last four or five weeks. I never saw that we were trudging toward Kevin's last days. Still, I've seen so many sick people that I knew in my heart what was happening. Kevin was not going to be in that coveted group of cancer survivors. Something made him buy our daughters' birthday presents early. This was out of character for him, but I didn't see it. I didn't want to see it.

Kevin complained of pain near one of his ribs, so he endured another round of scans. The results were sent to the wrong place, and for a month we couldn't get them. Everyone on Kevin's care team tried to track down the documents, including me.

What we didn't know was that the cancer had metastasized. It had invaded other places in his body. If the doctor had known that, Kevin's aggressive medical treatment would have ended instantly. They would have known the cancer was too widespread for the treatment to be effective. Instead, they would have initiated a palliative care philosophy. The doctor would have told us nothing could stop the cancer's progression. Instead, they would have worked to make Kevin as comfortable as possible as the cancer took his life.

MEMENTOS

My daughters would have liked something personal from their dad in his handwriting. He wasn't a big writer and could barely write in cursive, so he practiced his handwriting before he wrote anything important. He often wrote out what he wanted to say on the back of an envelope or old grocery list. Years after Kevin died, I found an envelope that he used to practice a birthday message to one of the girls. Although I had it laminated, the other daughter will never have an envelope of her own. I wish someone had told Kevin to write notes to the kids.

TUBE FEEDING

Kevin couldn't rely on his swallowing because of the size and location of the tumor, so the doctors put a GI feeding tube into his stomach. He would choke when he tried to eat and cough up saliva, called aspiration. That saliva goes back into the lungs and can cause pneumonia.

Tube feeding is terrible. It was one of the worst parts of witnessing Kevin's decline. The cancer process naturally reduces the appetite. The body protects itself by eating less. Tube feeding is a type of forced feeding.

It's an incredibly vulnerable position to be in. We were not given the opportunity to talk about the tube feeding. We didn't know that hundreds of different types of formula are available. We didn't know what questions to ask.

chapter eight
planning a funeral

In January, Kevin got really sick. I saw his blood reports every day, and his white blood cell count was far too low. I didn't think he would live much longer based on his blood work and his limited activity. He couldn't do anything—he wouldn't even turn the television on. He just sat in his recliner, pulling his energy back into himself. By then he could barely keep his eyes open. He needed help getting out of the chair and back into bed. Since he'd lost so much weight, he was cold all the time. My daughter often retrieved his heather-gray old-man sweater that zipped from the bottom and the top so we could easily get it on him.

Kevin loved that sweater. He wore it all the time, even to bed, along with his Philadelphia Eagles hat because he couldn't get warm.

Everybody in our community knew Kevin was going through cancer treatment. We started receiving a lot of get-well cards, Padre Pio cards, vials of holy water, prayer blankets, and other religious trinkets.

And we received many gifts aimed at keeping him warm—blankets and heated slippers.

I planned for his survival. I filled out the paperwork for his long-term disability, because we knew that when the radiation was done, Kevin wouldn't have much of a voice. I also planned for his death. The blood work results, paired with the decline I saw in his ability to function, made me think I'd better be prepared.

Planning a funeral was not something I had experience doing, and I thought really hard about which funeral home to pick. I didn't want the kids to be traumatized driving past it all the time. My parents came to help me. We told everyone we were going to lunch. They put me in the back seat of their car, and I cried the entire way to the funeral home.

The building was white with black shutters. I met Judi, the woman who would become Kevin's funeral director. She was wonderful and explained all of the decisions I needed to make. Did I want an open casket? Glasses on or off? Shoes? There's no way Kevin would go without his beloved sneakers. What clothes would he wear? My favorite green polo shirt that always made his green eyes pop—and khaki pants, of course.

Would Kevin be buried, entombed, or cremated? If buried, he would need to be embalmed. He would need a casket and a grave site. If cremated, he wouldn't need those things. Instead, all he would need was a simple pine box with a cardboard lid and an urn. I could spend anywhere from $80 to $4,000 on an urn. Should I ask his parents or siblings for input? And what about the cost? Who would pay for it?

They really did have pine boxes like you'd expect from the old days—plain, unadorned, and smooth to the touch. As the price increased, the quality did, too. The wood choices changed from pine to cherry. As the price raised, the scratchy linen casket lining became soft with beautiful stitching. I could buy a casket for Kevin that cost $30,000 or the simple box for $780.

Either way, I needed something to transport Kevin's remains to the funeral home and later to the church. For an open casket funeral service, he'd need to be embalmed. I chose cremation and an urn. I also bought him a really fabulous casket. I knew he would like the darker oak wood. I also chose it for how the liner felt. It was very soft.

There was even cremation jewelry I could buy, including necklaces I could fill with ashes and wear around. I bought the girls necklaces but had no plans to put ashes in them, just flowers or pictures. Judi was so respectful while I made these horrible decisions.

To Kevin and the girls, I kept my game face on, "Go team! Beat this cancer!" But I also had to take care of myself and plan for the reality facing us.

Kevin had already completed his advance directives for his job. I knew that if he was still alive but couldn't speak for himself, he didn't want to be on a ventilator. He didn't want to be kept alive artificially.

I called our town hall to let them know a sick person lived in our house. That way when it snowed, they would send the plow to our street early to make sure the area was clear for an emergency. The fire department did a walk-through of our home in case they needed to take him out quickly. They instructed me to keep a Do Not Resuscitate Order form on the fridge. It was a florescent pink sheet of paper with instructions about Kevin's code status, which told the emergency workers what his treatment wishes were—no CPR, no extreme measures to save his live. If they found Kevin dead, they would not use extraordinary measures to bring him back.

MARRIAGE

After Kevin died, more than one woman told me she wished her husband had died instead of mine. I know not every marriage is good, but if you don't like your marriage that much, get out. What if your husband gets sick? What would you be willing to do for him? What if you were ill?

JOY

What you feel ebbing away. What you wonder if you'll ever feel again.

chapter nine

reconnection

I worked as long as I could, until I couldn't stand it anymore. While I longed to be with Kevin, I wanted to be as far away from the sickness as possible. I never acclimated to the shock of seeing Kevin's body deteriorate. I was terrified of what was happening inside. He'd always struggled to lose weight, and now I could see his ribs. His face looked different because the cancer pushed out on one side, making his face look asymmetrical.

On the outside I was calm, but inside I screamed constantly. I couldn't cry. I had to put my feelings into a compartment where the sadness and fear couldn't get out. My shoulders shook with unshed tears.

It was the first Tuesday in March. Up until that point, I'd attended every single one of Kevin's appointments. But on this day, I was due to return to work. I dropped him off right in front of the cancer center doors and waited until he made it inside. I cried the entire drive in. The minute my co-worker walked into my office, I started bawling again.

This woman was not known for overwhelming expressions of compassion, but she went to the HR person and the office manager and told them I needed seven weeks off. All of my patient visits were canceled, save the first one with a young woman.

"You're pregnant and due in November," I said, sharing the happy news.

All I could think about was Kevin. I was afraid he'd be long dead by the time this woman's baby was born.

After I ushered her out, I drove back to the hospital with tears in my eyes. I reported to the receptionist in the cancer center, who told me to go right to the cancer suite. I walked down that tunnel of a hallway with my heels clicking on the floor. No employees were in sight. Every exam room door was open, and I peeked in each one as I walked by. Nope, not that one, that's the turban lady. Nope, not the one with the old guy's feet.

Suddenly, I saw Kevin in the last room straight ahead. I walked faster. He sat with his head down, looking at his sneakers. He still wore his green Philadelphia Eagles jacket and the Eagles hat he always wore.

He heard me and looked up with an expression of such joyous recognition and pure relief that I knew immediately I'd made the right choice. My old job was over. My new job had begun. From that moment on, I would be a full-time advocate, caretaker, comforter, GI tube feeder, dressing changer, medicine passer, pulse taker, and nagger.

I'd promoted myself to providing care at the bedside or beside the recliner, where I would crouch on my knees in supplication, prayerful caregiving, and silent begging.

Instead of checking in with colleagues, I would bargain with a higher power.

Please let me be strong. Please don't let me hurt him. Please don't let him see me crying. Please let me comfort him. Don't let him puke. Don't let him be cranky. Please don't let him ask me questions I don't know the answers to.

When I stopped working, we started gazing at each other again. We were side-by-side, and any stress from the tough times in our marriage just melted away. Words became less important. Presence was the most important thing. We couldn't touch, but we were connected in a physical way just having our bodies in the same room, our eyes locked on each other.

At times he cried in frustration, in pain, in uncertainty. Other times he was unreasonable, asking the same questions over and over again, cranky with me and the kids. Some days, when nothing went well, it was my fault. Early on, I argued back and defended myself.

"Well no, you bastard, the bills did not get paid because you were in the hospital. I was there all hours because you wanted me there, although I'm still not sure why."

The chemo brain. I wish he hadn't had it at the end.

I think he wanted me there because he loved me and trusted me. Things were all right if I said they were. I could make small talk and read from the newspaper and be there when he woke up. More than once, my presence got him better care. Word spread quickly that I was a nurse—maybe it helped, maybe it didn't. I hoped it did help.

The home care nurse came to the house to deliver the chemotherapy. I debated whether it was a godsend or an intrusion. Kevin's chemo had to be disconnected every Saturday evening, usually around 6:00 p.m. Every time the nurse came, I cleaned up and got the house ready. But the nurse always showed up late—with a forced cheerfulness and familiarity that made me uncomfortable. I didn't want her to think that things were less than perfect. I didn't want to be the lady with the messy house on top of everything else.

I always offered coffee and fresh warm cookies. She always accepted and pulled up a chair to chat. After half an hour or so, she opened her bag and prepared to change out the IV tubing. Every time, the nurse found she was missing something essential—gauze, tubing, a stethoscope. It was terrible.

I was a lunatic. Nobody cared what the house looked like, but it was one of the few things I could control. I should have left the house or taken a shower or looked at a book. Instead, I made sure the place was tidy, smelled good, and was welcoming. At least until you got upstairs to the makeshift hospital room, where the fifty-two-inch television stood. I'd given Kevin that awesome, overwhelming, guilt-ridden gift to make the time pass faster, to sleep in front of, to make noise and block noise. It was Kevin's soothing sedative. And mine, too—no need to talk, no need to think, just pass the remote control.

One day, we stopped on the way home from chemo at the local jewelry store. I called in advance to prepare them for our visit. I knew in my heart Kevin wasn't doing well. He was so sick and frail. When we stepped up into the store from the cobblestone sidewalk, the young, blond sales attendant led us beneath brick arches and past glittering cases to a small back room. Kevin wanted to pick out a special gift for the girls. His brain had slowed down, so she patiently showed him the array of beautiful jewelry set out in the back room.

"This one. And these," he said, pointing at a necklace and ring for each of our daughters. "I want them engraved."

He refused to leave me out, so the rings bore the message: "Love Dad and Mom." After we made our purchases, we headed to the car and passed a display of rings. My eye caught on a lovely diamond anniversary ring. We talked about it on the way home and agreed to buy it since our twenty-fifth wedding anniversary was that October. It was the first anniversary gift he'd ever purchased that far in advance.

When we talked, we remembered the good times and looked through pictures of us and our children when we were all younger.

Other times, we sat in silent desperation, wanting to understand the truth, trying to grasp the awfulness and the permanence of this absurd situation. I would have thrown myself down for all three members of my family, always. I'd never had to do that for Kevin, but the moment we discovered the cancer, I became territorial and protective of him. I didn't think Kevin would ever leave me. I thought we would die together.

EXIT STRATEGY

I am a big Plan B person, but I let that slip away during Kevin's treatment. I couldn't think about anything else when I was so heavily involved in Plan A. I felt like I couldn't take a moment away from the battle we were fighting. But at least we had our wills, financial planning, and advance directives in order. That helped tremendously. Those things became a parachute, so I could plan for a soft landing. While you're enjoying your life, plan for the end so the landing isn't harder than it needs to be.

HOSPICE AND PALLIATIVE CARE

Hospice philosophy is an acknowledgement that nothing more can be done to prolong life—no surgery, radiation, or chemo. The goal of medical care becomes providing care and comfort. Medical aggression isn't appropriate anymore.

Palliative care is a new branch of medicine that focuses on people diagnosed with a life-limiting or terminal illness. The palliative care nurse is an expert at talking to people. We see all the information on a patient's chart. We spend time with a patient. Palliative care specialists look at the whole picture. I didn't become a hospice and palliative care nurse practitioner until after Kevin's death. The hospice doctor who attended Kevin introduced me to the field and mentored my education.

A palliative care specialist would have looked at all of Kevin's charts and made sure we really took in the truth about Kevin's condition. Kevin was going to die prematurely one way or the other. The cancer would eventually take his life. A palliative care clinician would have helped us make truly informed decisions.

chapter ten
is this a love story?

I don't know if ours was a love story. We had a great time. We had a real marriage, made up of arguments, fun, daily moments of connection, and physical touch. There were times of disconnection and times we made up. He was the father of my children. My friend.

My definition of love was putting the other person first, their needs first. But I went too far. I never put myself first. In the early years, we'd work through our problems. But as time went on, we stopped fixing things after an argument. We each had wounds that hadn't healed.

In the last five years of his life, Kevin was less satisfied with his career and more pressured at work. Perhaps both of us were a little bored. We didn't make time for pleasure or to recharge our batteries.

The early years were all about building. Career building, family building. We loved to move around. We'd called this small town our home since 1989. We were probably ready for a change of scenery, but that's not what you do when you have kids. So we snapped at one another and argued. Things were not right.

At the same time, we talked repeatedly about the future.

"When we retire, we'll have time for each other. We'll travel again."

Somewhere along the way, our marriage settled into a general feeling of dissatisfaction. We used to have a rule: You can't leave the room angry. I wasn't good at anger, but Kevin was great at it. He could have been a lawyer. One day, I stood on the bottom of the stairs while he stood at the top. We yelled at each other, but he broke one of our fighting rules and stormed down the hall.

I no longer remember what that fight was about, though it was certainly important at the time. If I had to guess, I'd say it was about the kids. About letting the girls stay out too late, or homework left undone, or who was spoiling them. We fought, but we refused to talk about it.

The next day, Kevin called me up like nothing had happened. A part of our relationship was all business. He would call me every day the moment he left work, and we would talk throughout his entire drive home. I knew the people he worked with and he'd ask me for advice, and then he'd help me navigate my own job. We hung up each evening as I heard the garage door go up.

At the end, all of the anger and disconnection between us melted away. We made amends. We remembered each other. It was normal again.

And maybe that was love. Maybe love was that we knew each other in a way that we didn't have to use a lot of words. We didn't have to explain or introduce ourselves all the time. I knew who Kevin was. And I knew he knew me.

We lost each other sometimes, but I always knew he put me first. Always. People even commented on our connection. We were well married. He was the perfect choice for me. Was that love?

The bedroom Kevin and I shared stretched above the two-car garage. At the end was a rounded dormer window that let beautiful light into the room. One day in the middle of March, I fell asleep on my daughter's bed. In a lucid dream, I stood in front of that gorgeous window. Suddenly, a white dove crashed into it. I snapped awake. Instantly I knew what the dream was—a harbinger of death.

STAGES OF THE BODY SHUTTING DOWN

As the body shuts down, the dying person loses the ability to swallow. The muscles stop working. Theoretically, this is a protective measure. If the patient has trouble breathing, the body doesn't want the belly full of food because it takes blood away from the brain and heart. Saliva stays in the throat and causes a gurgling sound every time the patient breathes. Those secretions bother us more than the patients. If it bothered the patients, they would cough the saliva up. The secretions and sounds cause families a great deal of distress, and we treat those symptoms mostly for their benefit.

The gurgling breath is correlated with the stage of coma the person is in—at this point in the process, there is nothing anybody can do. It is part of dying. Usually the secretions indicate that the patient is essentially brain dead and has about twelve hours left before their heart stops.

Mottling is when parts of the body change color because of a change in circulation. The heart becomes too weak to pump blood to the distant extremities, such as the hands, feet, throat, and brain. The body shuts down from the outside in, and the blood is reserved for the organs in the core. Mottling often starts at the toes. The medical staff usually notices it by the time it reaches the ankles. From there it goes to the mid-calf, knee, and mid-thigh.

Anasarka is another part of dying. Because the kidneys shut down, people can swell up and their skin can split. The vessels lose their elasticity. By the time that happens, the patient is in such a deep coma that they don't feel anything. It becomes a temptation for families to think, "Let's try dialysis." But this kind of swelling occurs outside the vessels, so dialysis will not help.

PAIN

In the *Textbook of Basic Nursing,* by Caroline Bunker Rosdahl and Mary T. Kowalski, the authors report: "Margo McCaffery's definition of pain as 'whatever the experiencing person says it is, existing whenever and wherever the person says it does' has become the prevailing conceptualization of pain for clinicians over the past few decades."

I had expected Kevin to say he had more pain than he did, but he didn't like the way medications made him feel. He even had root canals done without Novocain. He took his first pain medication on the day before he died. He asked me to apply a Fentanyl patch for him because he was too weak to open the medication packet. The patch was a good choice for Kevin, since doctors expected he would have more problems swallowing as his disease and the treatment progressed.

The patch takes up to eighteen hours for the body to absorb the medication. We didn't know that. Other types of cancer can produce more pain. In pain control, a long-acting medication is usually given twice a day to keep the pain in the background. This way the person can keep participating in the activities of daily life. Cancer patients often experience "breakthrough" pain that comes on quickly and for no apparent reason. This pain is treated with a quick-acting medication, usually given in liquid form, to provide fast relief.

It is important to know the level of pain a patient is comfortable tolerating. We use a zero-to-ten scale, with zero being no pain and ten being the worst pain you can imagine.

Remember that pain medications have side effects, including sedation and constipation. People will shake off the sedation in about three days, but the constipation is ongoing. A bowel regimen will also be prescribed.

I was afraid of morphine. I thought it would hasten Kevin's death. Now I know that in the small doses used in hospice care, morphine relieves pain and the sensation of air hunger in the brain. It eases the work of breathing, so Kevin didn't burn up essential energy overexerting his muscles. It enabled him to breathe more comfortably.

chapter eleven
the final weekend

"This is all going to be over by Wednesday." It was Friday morning while we each made our beds. I thought I heard him correctly, but wasn't sure. I looked up at him and our eyes met.

"What?" I asked. Kevin was obviously upset. His gravelly voice, destroyed by the radiation, broke, and he kept stopping as though considering what he was about to say.

As I walked over to him, he said it again. "This will all be over." We stepped into a silent hug.

I knew what he was really saying, but part of me thought, *Oh, he's talking about this intense treatment. This portion will be over soon.* Kevin admitted for the first time that day that he felt pain. Weeks before, the doctor gave me a pain patch to apply to his skin, which I did after Kevin said he was hurting. I didn't know it took eighteen hours for the medication to hit his blood stream, so he suffered in silence while we hustled to get to his radiation appointment.

That day he needed a CAT scan to assess how the treatment was going. Since he was allergic to the dye used in the procedure, he needed to take a lot of medicine before the scan—steroids, Benedryl, antacids, anti-nausea pills. The drugs made him so tired.

When he left the waiting room for radiation treatment, I couldn't go with him. During the treatment he wore a mask on his face, like a hockey mask with an onion-netting pattern on it, which the nurses screwed down to the table so he couldn't move. He just hated it. He would get really nauseous. Sometimes he took an anxiety drug to take the edge off, and that made him tired, too.

Everything ran on schedule that day. Still, we stayed for several extra hours since he needed the long version of the CAT scan. After returning from the radiation, he had to take the dye for the scan. By the end of it all, Kevin was completely exhausted.

"We should check in and try to talk to the doctor today," I said.

"No, I just want to go home," he said. "I'm really tired."

We stayed at the cancer center a few minutes to see if he would change his mind and check in.

"No," he repeated. "I want to go home." The nurse told me to put six cups of water through the feeding tube to flush the dye. I said I'd do it.

He sat in the passenger seat of his Suburban while I drove. His favorite green jacket puffed up around his small frame—it was at least three sizes too big. He leaned back heavily against the headrest.

As we drove home down Central Avenue, Kevin was silent. I talked for both of us. In my practiced caregiver's monologue, I replayed and reinforced the day's actions because it helped Kevin feel less stress. "Get up, brush your teeth, do you have to go to the bathroom?"

I always drilled ahead, even planning the route to and from the cancer center because Kevin got so anxious.

"You're going to go the same way, right?" he would ask. "You're not going to take a short cut, right? You're not going to get behind a school bus, are you?" And I would get irritated.

On this trip home he remained quiet, so I told him my strategy for flushing fluids through him. I told him he could just rest. I assured him the nurse thought his fatigue was from the Benedryl. They'd given him a huge dose.

About a mile from home, Kevin spoke. "Fill up the tank with gas," he said.

"But it's not empty," I replied, thinking, *I don't want to take the time to do that. You're tired. I want to get you home.* I glanced at him. Taking in the sight of his wasted body, I pulled into the gas station beneath the tall black sign with its starburst of green. It was the most expensive gas station in town, with service that included personalized help cleaning your windshield.

I watched as the gas attendant used his squeegee to create long rows of beaded, dripping grime that he cleaned with precise, squeaking swipes. It was a marvel. I didn't think the windshield was even dirty, but now I could see through it clearly.

I wish I could have seen my husband's illness as clearly.

Reaching into the back seat, I grabbed two twenties out of my purse. Kevin rolled his head toward me. He flicked irritation at me with his eyes, speaking in the silent language of long-married couples. I knew what he was thinking.

"It's more than twenty dollars. Use the card, since we get one percent money back with every purchase."

I slipped the credit card out of my wallet and, after the attendant rapped on my window, handed it over.

"Forty dollars," he said.

I had pulled that exact amount of cash out of my wallet. Just a few short weeks ago, we would have laughed our heads off. Kevin would have ribbed me about always spending cash. I would have reminded him of my physic abilities. It would have been one of those moments that a marriage is made of. *I remember you.*

We pulled up in front of Kevin's dream house. His appearance worried me. He looked so tired, and his skin was paler than usual. "I'm going to take you through the front door so you can go right up the stairs," I said, instead of taking him on our usual route through the garage.

I helped him take his jacket off, and he dropped heavily into the recliner. I thought it was strange that he didn't go to the bathroom. Usually he would go before he rested, but not this time. I didn't ask him about it. I put his feet up and covered him in a gray blanket with the Philadelphia Eagles logo on it. They were his favorite team. He still wore his sneakers. He loved his sneakers and always wore the same pair. I covered his feet with a prayer shawl the people from our church gave us. Then I took his glasses off and set them in a tray beside the chair. He was that tired. He fell asleep right away.

I followed the nurse's instructions, putting water into the feeding tube while he slept. *One more caregiving chore complete.*

The house was somewhat clean, and we had a few hours before Christine was due home from school. I was so tired—my bones, my soul, my heart were so tired. I decided to lie down. Not for long. I didn't mean to rest for long.

I settled on top of our bed and sunk into the comforter with a book. I was so comfortable and warm and pleased that Kevin slept. I woke up at about 2:30 or 3:00 p.m. Kevin was still asleep. He hadn't changed position. Quietly, I picked up the phone to call my mother.

"He's sleeping now. I'm not going to wake him. I'll let him rest a little longer. He looks so peaceful," I told her. I dozed off again. I woke up with a shock at around 4:00 p.m. And it just hit me. *Something's wrong.*

I'd been so relieved he was peaceful, but all of a sudden it didn't make sense anymore. I flew out of bed and tried to wake him up. I couldn't. He wouldn't wake up. I tried to control the screaming in my head, but it wouldn't stop.

Please, please not like this, not today.

What time is it? Where's Christine? When is she due home? What is happening? Why aren't you moving, and why are your sneakers still on? I hate those sneakers! You know you're supposed to take them off when you put your feet on the furniture and you usually take them off as soon as you walk in the door and I did not mean to fall asleep and the medicine is still in your system and you will be up soon.

Five more minutes. Please, please, just one minute.

Please say something to me. Please move. Open your eyes.

Why is your skin so cold and why does it feel so stiff like wax and oh my god your lips they're blue and you aren't moving and you're kidding me right?

One more second.

Say anything.

Say that you're all right and not in pain and not mad at me for letting my guard down. I told you I would be the nurse, but right now

I am every inch the wife and so sorry I agreed to be the nurse and please can we do this over?

Please. Talk to me. There's one more thing I want to ask you. I don't know how to do this and I can't remember anything and how did we get here? Can you please wake up?

Kevin still had a pulse. His chest rose with each soft breath. I called the hospice nurse, the doctor, and my friend Marge, who was also a hospice nurse. Once the calls were made, I slumped on the edge of the bed and stared at my husband.

The voice in my mind berated me. *How could you have missed this coming? How stupid can you possibly be?*

Marge arrived first. She called my family, his family. My parents drove from their home in Rhode Island and picked up Katie from college. I still thought he would snap out of it. I mean, we did everything right. This was the wrong ending.

My daughter Christine came home from high school. Because she didn't really understand what was happening, she treated him like he was just napping. She popped in and out of his room. We read. We watched TV. Then Katie and my parents arrived.

Kevin was still in the recliner. It didn't occur to us to move him. He looked okay. He was sleeping. I didn't know if it was the medication or if he was in a coma, but the more time went by, the more it looked like Kevin was in a coma. He had a pulse and good circulation, but he was non-responsive. Nobody knew what direction he would go in. At about 9:00 p.m., the hospice doctor said, "We'll know more in the morning."

Weeks before, Kevin made me promise I would not take him back to the hospital for overnight treatment. Early on, he was delighted to go to the hospital because he felt safe and monitored by the professionals. As his illness progressed, he wanted to stay home, and I honored that. He stayed home, and the hospice nurses came to us. I stopped providing the care. I tried to keep everybody posted about his condition and was in constant contact with our parents and our children. I made it look easy. Just like Kevin knew I would. The shock was my armor, and I used it well.

Katie slept on the small table right next to her father. I fell asleep listening to Kevin's breathing. It sounded normal, with the occasional gentle snore. I slept through the night.

In the morning, things were the same, which meant Kevin was actually much worse. Even though he looked the same, he hadn't moved or gone to the bathroom. I don't remember who took off Kevin's sneakers, but it wasn't me. Instead he wore warm slippers and the same two warm blankets. Although he appeared comfortable, his body was shutting down. He wasn't going to get better.

I knew just by looking at Kevin that his spirit was long gone. He hadn't moved in eighteen hours. The nurse came over again, and I called his parents and told them what was happening. The whole day was so surreal. People stopped over all day, including church friends, co-workers, and the kids' friends. My mother was there the whole time. She buzzed around with a tray of hot and cold drinks and snacks.

Marge and my dad sat vigil. I didn't. I couldn't. I wouldn't. I ran around like a lunatic. I drove Christine to rehearsal, I vacuumed, I ran errands—nomadic in my grief.

I wish I could say the day was orchestrated, but it wasn't. People just knew what to do. Nobody interfered with anybody else. There was more laughter than tears.

My father picked Christine up from rehearsal. And on his way to the school, he drove in the wrong exit in a small act of rebellion that he and the kids still talk about.

When they got home, the hospice nurse sat everybody down.

"There have been changes," she said. Kevin's breathing had slowed and become shallow. His heart rate had slowed as well. His skin color turned a dusky grayish purple. We watched Kevin's favorite movie on that giant television. It was about the Philadelphia Eagles, their history and the players. He and the kids loved watching it, so I left and rested a bit. People were in and out. It was so normal, like having a backyard barbecue. No crying. No hysterics.

At about 4:00 p.m., his breathing became much more labored and raspy. I could hear his breathing, and see him throw his shoulders up as he struggled for air. It was hard to watch. The nurse suggested giving him liquid morphine. She explained that it would ease the work of breathing and reduce the sensation of air hunger in his brain. The nurse put just a few drops of morphine under his tongue. His breathing relaxed, and he stopped jerking his shoulders. The medication helped him conserve energy. He looked more comfortable.

Marge's partner, Ann, and her friend Judy came by. It was around quarter to five and everybody was hungry for supper, so we ordered a bunch of Chinese food. Ann and Judy set up the meal on the breakfast bar in the kitchen. It was like a New Year's Eve buffet. It was an occasion. People got cold drinks, sat down at the table, chatted. They took turns visiting Kevin.

Upstairs, Kevin continued to decline. His body felt ice cold, and his skin looked purple. I knew what was coming. Soon. Not right then, but soon. He had a lot of saliva, so now he made a gurgling sound when he breathed—a clear sign the end was coming. The nurse repositioned him and that helped. The next dose of morphine helped, too.

It's so hard to die, I thought. *But you make it look effortless.*

Kevin's sister and her husband arrived. Around 7:30 p.m., the snow started falling: a thick, bright white snow. The kids were up and down the stairs. They settled in the living room downstairs and watched reruns of Saturday Night Live. Their laughter filled the house. Marge planned to stay the night, but my parents decided to go back to the hotel at 11:00 p.m. since the snow continued to pile up. Before people left for the night, we gathered around Kevin's bed for a prayer service with Kevin's family, a retired minister, my parents, my children, and my friends. We sang *Amazing Grace.* Then everybody started clearing out.

My parents gathered their belongings.

"Honey, I need a drop in my eye. Would you mind helping me?" my mother asked. She could never put in eye drops herself. We walked together to the bathroom, and we talked and laughed a bit. The kids were still downstairs laughing their heads off. I put the drop in my mother's eye, and as I brought my hand down, one of the cats screamed. I let go of the dropper and turned to the hallway. I headed to the right to find out what happened to the cats, Chip and Mick. My dad came toward me from the left. I thought he was coming to see what was wrong with the cats, too, but he just stopped.

"Lynn," he said. And again. "Lynn." It was one of those moments when time stopped. Suddenly I knew. I couldn't hear Kevin's breathing anymore.

Since he'd gone into a coma, I'd timed my breathing to his. Sometimes he panted, and other times it was like a long exhale, with ten or twenty seconds between every breath. I couldn't hear it anymore. And my dad didn't have to say anything. He took me by the arm, just above my elbow, and we walked the half dozen steps down the hall together. Kevin sat in the chair and he looked fine. He wasn't purple anymore. He wasn't waxy anymore. His skin even had a bit of give to it.

Marge wore my stethoscope around her neck, and she had her sweater pulled up on her forearm. She stared at her watch.

What's my stethoscope doing around your neck? I thought it was so strange.

"I listened for a full minute, and there's no more heartbeat," Marge said. Then she broke down. My mom and dad, we all cried. I'd never seen my parents cry.

I could still hear the kids laughing. *I don't want to tell them,* I thought.

When the girls came upstairs, they lost it. They were hysterical, screaming and crying. They kept moving from one adult to the next for a hug or the right word, but there was no comfort.

My father called the funeral home. I didn't know what to do. I didn't want Kevin's body in the house for long. It was late. We were tired and sad, and the kids were crazy with grief. I didn't want them to have the death scene in their heads, so I sent them to the living room where they wouldn't be able to see the funeral home attendants taking their father out of the house for the last time.

When Judi, our funeral director and her employees showed up, they took Kevin out of the recliner. He wore khaki pants and a pajama shirt that had fallen askew. I adjusted it for him. They had trouble getting him down the stairs because of the angle, but eventually they took him downstairs and to the front door, with the body bag zipped up to his neck so I could see his face.

It was still snowing. "Please. Cover his face," I said. I didn't want the cold snowflakes touching him. Judi ever so gently pulled the zipper up all the way. I could see the lines in the snow where the gurney had rolled, but thankfully, I couldn't see the hearse. I didn't want to see them drive down the street, taking Kevin away.

My dad shut the door.

I'm so tired. I'll always be this tired, I thought.

We joined the kids at the back of the house.

"It was 11:11 when he died," my mother said.

The girls thought it was magical since 11:11 was in the lyrics to one of their favorite songs, "Konstantine" by Something Corporate. "It's 11:11. And now you want to talk."

We all went to bed a few minutes later. The girls cried themselves to sleep. I crawled into the small guest bed down the hall. *I'm not going to get over this,* I thought.

I never slept in our marital bed again.

Sunday morning, I began arranging things to stay as busy as possible. I booked hotel rooms and called the maids to come clean the house. I threw the sheets from our bed into the washer and dryer, and then back in the washer again, and back and forth so many times I lost count. Then I just threw them away. I threw away the cleanest sheets in the world.

I didn't want people in the house because I didn't want a lot of negative energy around. No one was staying with us, thankfully. I couldn't take care of anyone else right then. It was just me and the kids. People stopped by with food and flowers. We hugged, but no one came through the door.

During the day, I went upstairs to lie down. My mom checked on me, but even though I was wide awake, I shut my eyes and pretended I was sleeping so I wouldn't have to talk.

It was such a shock to me that Kevin died. *I felt like an idiot.* That last Friday, I was so happy he could rest peacefully. I never thought he'd started his journey to eternal rest. The clinician in me had checked out, and that day I was just Kevin's wife. I missed the whole thing. It wasn't what I wanted. I was shocked. No. Horrified. The missing was an ache, a void that I knew I could never fill back up. And soon, I wouldn't be able to hold back the monstrous grief I'd held at bay the last three months.

Give me five more minutes with him. I'm not ready for this. Just five more minutes, I prayed. While he was still alive, we were pummeled constantly with bad news and awful decisions to make. I thought about the water I'd put down his feeding tube. *Did his bladder get full? Did I hurt him? Where did all that water go?*

WITNESSING DEATH

If your spouse is still alive, or if you're feeling guilty or upset that you didn't witness his last breath, this is for you: You don't have to stand there and watch him die. In fact, seventy percent of the time, husbands and wives don't want to die in front of each other. The dying person will pass the moment the spouse goes to the bathroom or leaves to grab a cup of coffee. It's very common. And that's what happened to me. If you want to sit with your loved one the entire time, do. If you don't want to, don't feel badly that you can't sit still.

BLAME

After Kevin died, I made appointments with his oncologist and radiologist. His death was too sudden. I thought we had more time. I wanted to understand how this had happened. You have every right to visit the doctors after the fact to answer any unanswered questions. When a patient has both chemotherapy and radiation therapy, there are two different departments, two different doctors, and two sets of staff. You check in one place and come out and go check in at the second place. There are two sets of charts.

In September, I spoke to a lawyer about possibly suing Kevin's primary care physician, the one who prescribed allergy medications instead of a visit to the ear, nose, and throat specialist. Kevin had gone in to see his doctor five times that final year, but the doctor missed the cancer. His dentist missed it. I wonder: If I had been the nurse practitioner working on Kevin's case, would I have missed it? It was far back on his tonsil and hard to see, but the weight loss and night sweats were clues, hallmarks of cancer. I wanted answers.

How could this have happened?

So many treatments in the medical profession are done as if the doctor is reading from a cookbook. If this treatment fails, try that. When that one fails, try something else.

The profession sets us up to assume that a patient's death is a treatment failure, that it was somebody's fault. We need to fix this kind of thinking. People die. We all do. Kevin died of complications from cancer. You can't get stuck thinking that somebody else dropped the ball, or you'll never feel free to move on.

chapter twelve

saying goodbye

On Monday, my brother-in-law called the oncologist's office.

"Hi," he said. "Kevin Devlin won't be coming in. He doesn't need your services anymore." A laugh escaped his lips, and as he hung up, we both laughed until we cried. I walked upstairs and switched the computer on. The tears flowed. *So much water. Where does it all come from?*

I had a job to do: Kevin's obituary. I knew I didn't want a photo because all I could think about was his face lining someone's cat litter box. I wrote a brief and to-the-point paragraph, with the time and date of the wake and funeral, and broke into sobs.

In many ways I was in shock. I couldn't believe he was gone. At the same time, I felt tremendous relief.

I don't have to take care of him anymore.

When the crying subsided, I called Christine's hairdresser and booked an appointment for my daughters and me the morning of the wake. All the busy work made me feel better—made me feel like I had something solid to hang on to.

There were no customers in the salon except for Katie, Christine, and me. The hairdressers worked like a bunch of bees in a hive. They acted like there was nothing else in the world to do but brush and style the kids' hair and blow mine out. They took such good care of us. We hadn't had any care or comfort during the last three months, none of us had. And those women helped us so much, simply by taking us out of our grim reality for a few moments. We laughed and listened to music. It was the first time we'd been out of the house as a group, the three of us, in a long time.

As I watched my girls getting primped, it struck me that the three of us were formally preparing to meet the world as a new unit—one without a husband or a father. We practiced telling our story to those kind women and began learning how to accept condolences.

At some point, I started shaking badly. I think my body needed a place for the stress hormones to go.

Visiting hours at the funeral home were 2:00 to 4:00 p.m. and 6:00 to 8:00 p.m. People typically go home between the two sessions, but I didn't want to leave Kevin. I'd told the florist I didn't want any lilies because I'd never liked how they smelled and none of the bouquets in our designated room included them. Even the stray lilies that made it into the funeral home didn't make it past Judi, who pulled them all out.

I brought bags of slippers, Gatorade, and Fig Newtons because so many people were traveling in. I knew they'd be hungry and standing on their feet a long time. To be a nurse, you have to be a caretaker. I had the caretaker gene in spades, sometimes to my own detriment.

But now I took comfort in doing these things for other people. It gave me something to do.

One more caretaking chore checked off.

The casket was strategically placed against the wall at the front of the room with chairs lined up beside it. My co-workers were in the back line of chairs. I had assigned them to act like bouncers to protect my kids. I didn't want anyone saying a hurtful or inappropriate comment to my girls.

When I wasn't shaking people's hands, I sat in the front row with my parents, Katie, Christine, and Kevin's parents.

Christine's friends from school came and I didn't make her stand there visiting with people. She was only fifteen and couldn't handle it. Katie wouldn't leave. She wanted every hand shake, every hug. The girls played music from mixes they'd created from Kevin's favorites.

At the break, everybody gathered in their clans. His parents, brothers, and sisters went one place, and my parents took my kids out for a while.

Between the two wakes, after everyone had left, I stayed. The thought of leaving Kevin alone was unbearable to me. I sat alone next to his coffin and visited with him for two hours. I hadn't seen him for twenty-four hours, and he looked so peaceful and comfortable. He looked better than before because the unhealthy colors faded away after he died. The cancerous swelling on his face was completely gone.

Coffins are very wide, and I kept thinking I could climb in with him, but I didn't. I just sat next to him and cried and cried and cried. I dreaded the moment when they'd close the coffin for good.

There was no wastepaper basket nearby, so I dropped my used tissues on the carpet. Judi came in and saw me next to the coffin with balled-up tissues all over the floor. She went to find my sister. It was time for round two.

The funeral was on March 28, 2007, at 10:00 a.m. because Kevin and I had married at 10:00 a.m. We weren't late. It was important to not be late. I was always the late one, while Kevin had always arrived exactly on time wherever he went. From now on, in honor of Kevin, I would be punctual.

When we pulled into the parking lot of the Methodist church we'd attended for years, people stood waiting for us. Parked on one side was a school bus filled with high school kids in the jazz gospel choir.

Instead of flowers or a donation, a friend arranged for and paid to have our local sub shop make bag lunches for hundreds of people. So many travelers showed up, but not everybody could come to the reception and eat. The kids in the choir could only stay to perform their songs because they had to return to school to take tests. Kevin's co-workers at GE had to get back to punch the clock. Neither group would have time to eat lunch.

Kevin loved oversized spearmint Life Savers, and we provided them in his memory. Lots of them were left over, so my friend distributed them into the lunch bags. I was so glad she helped in this way, instead of cooking us a casserole we'd never eat.

I climbed out of the car, hoping my skirt was not above my butt. My friend handed me the eulogy I'd emailed her that morning. As I walked toward the church I'd spent so much time in with the kids and Kevin, I shook the whole way. Even the back of my legs were shaking. There was no one there to hold on to. My parents and children walked behind me, so I was alone. I didn't want to go in.

By the time I made it through the door and into the church, the mix of songs the girls made played over the loud speakers. Rupert Holmes sang about making love at midnight as I crossed the threshold. After that, Scottish music filled the hall. Kevin was already there waiting for me at the front, just like at our wedding.

I'd arranged to have small bottles of Gatorade beneath the first rows of pews just in case. I didn't know if my family remembered to eat or drink.

The choir sang *Pachelbel Canon in D* and *Amazing Grace*. People filled every row on the main floor and the balcony, too.

Soon it was my turn to take the podium. This is what I said:

> Good Morning. My family wants to thank you all for coming this morning and attending the wake yesterday. We are extremely touched by the kind words of sympathy and fond remembrances offered during this very terrible time. The online tributes are especially moving. Many of them refer to a story or anecdote that we knew something about because Kevin had shared it with us over dinner. It is so comforting to know that the man we knew and loved was the same man you all knew and loved.
>
> Kevin had a presence. He loved to talk, but he also knew how to listen. When Kevin was diagnosed with stage four cancer on December 1, 2006, we knew time was going to be short and the treatment would be intense. The specialist in Boston was quite clear that if the cancer did not take him, then the aggressive treatment could. To no one's surprise,

Kevin chose aggressive treatment and tolerated it without complaint.

I've been a nurse for just about ever and never understood why cancer was always referred to as a "battle" or why the patient was called a cancer "victim." I get it now. Cancer is a bully. It knows what it's going to do to you. It will flog you. It will kick you when you're down and in ways you never dreamed possible. But in Kevin's usual style, he never asked "why me?" In fact, he told me how we were going to handle the diagnosis. He said, "I don't really understand this medical thing, you handle that. I look at cancer as nothing more than a production problem, and I can fix a production problem."

I had the privilege of knowing Kevin for twenty-seven years. He was ours—Katie's, Christine's, and mine. He always put his family first. He was a wonderful example of a loving husband and father. From the loving presence we are surrounded by today, I realize I shared him with all of you.

When we first brought baby Katie home to our apartment in Pennsylvania, Kevin carried her through every room. He introduced her to her crib and every object in her room. Then he introduced her to the rest of the apartment. We stepped out onto the tiny balcony, and though I am firmly convinced that Katie was quite asleep in her Dad's arms, he introduced her to the trees and pointed out the local elementary school and other landmarks. After he completed the tour, he turned to me and said, "Now what?"

I guess that's my question for today. Now what?

And I can hear Kevin say, "Password protect everything! Every time you write a check, mark it in the book. Get a receipt for tax deductions. Fill up the car with gas."

Katie, Christine, and I will start a new life together, filled with Daddy-isms, and will have our whole lives to honor him as he honored us. Thank you, Kevin. Thank you for your every kindness. And thank you for our girls. We had a wonderful life together, and I will see you again.

We left his body at the front of the church and streamed toward the entrance. I didn't want the girls—or myself—to see the funeral home people close the casket or see the hearse drive away. I didn't want the kids throwing themselves over the coffin, which was a possibility. It was a lot of work keeping them propped up. They had expressed a lot of grief, and now it was time to stay strong.

Though the ceremony started slow and sad, by the end it was a celebration. *Celebrate Me Home* by Kenny Loggins played through the speakers. The rest of the crowd followed us outside and down a short path to the dining hall, where the church ladies had prepared a funeral luncheon. Kevin's co-workers stood outside and watched him go.

People sat and ate at tables spread throughout the room. Flowers decorated the front, where the tiled floor was clear for those who wanted to stand. Some people took flower arrangements home. Some went to our house. Church volunteers took the rest of the flowers to area nursing homes.

And then it was over. The months of fear, the shock and horror of watching the man I loved die. That part was over, and it gave me time to discover something: Our marriage was like a three-legged stool—me, Kevin, and our marriage. When I lost him, I lost two legs of the stool, the marriage and the man. A lot of my identity was tied up in my relationship with him. Marriage is about merging, so I never made an exit strategy.

After the guests left, the casseroles were discarded, and the dishes cleaned, I went to bed and hardly got out for months.

CONDOLENCES, FOOD, AND GIFTS

It's hard when someone says they're sorry for your loss. At first, you want to punch them in the face. Then the moment often turns and the person saying they're sorry wants you to comfort *them*. Since I was my husband's caregiver, I hadn't had any comfort at all for a long time. I was so used to taking care of everybody else that I automatically kept my needs to myself. Really, there was nothing anyone could say. I so desperately wanted a word of comfort, but nothing could take my pain away.

Still, people wanted to help, and I could accept some things better than others. Instead of a guest book, the funeral home helped us build a website that accepted online tributes to Kevin. Hundreds of people posted wonderful stories about him. We had them printed and bound into a lovely book. That worked for me. The cards were beautiful. A friend sent a card every week while Kevin was sick and for the entire year after his death. Flowers or edible arrangements are fantastic, casseroles are not.

This is going to sound harsh because I know people are simply doing their best, but the smell of food made me sick. After the casseroles were dropped off at my house, I put them all down the garbage disposal. Then I had to do all those dishes and remember who had given me which dish so I could return it.

The best gift I received was from a girlfriend who asked if she could take my daughter to a matinee. It wasn't for a long amount of time, which was good because we felt clingy for each other, but it was good for my daughter to go and chill—and good for me to have time to myself.

CHORES

The tasks of running a household are immense. No matter how much your spouse didn't do around the house, it soon becomes apparent that you were a team. The chores he did were immeasurable and invaluable. You have to decide, and rather quickly, how much of his work you can take on. Don't succumb to being a martyr. Think about selling the house. You need time to take care of yourself and your family without doing all the chores your spouse once did, too.

chapter thirteen
the soggy year

So many people attended the funeral. The business types shook my hand, mumbled something about being sorry for my loss, and said, "Call if there's anything I can do." They told stories about Kevin extending what he thought was an everyday kindness but to them stood out as being extraordinary—saving a job, restoring a shift, working over Christmas. He was one of the "guys": a real boss and mentor, a smart guy, a company man. He knew the history of the business and cared about its future. He was a moral compass, they said.

After they shook my hand or hugged me, they grasped my right hand in their right hand and smacked me on the left upper arm, as if to complete a secret handshake or code. They weren't trying to hurt me, but one of my office managers whispered, "They have to stop hitting you." She could hear the sound of their palms slapping my arm. The next day my upper arm ached. I lifted up the sleeve of my favorite silk blouse and there was a bruise, green and purple and blue. There it was, proof that something terrible had happened to our family.

People in our community called the girls and me courageous, tough, and strong. All we wanted to do was lay down and scream and cry and protest. We made it through, but were so raw and bruised.

After Kevin died, people brought us things. They dropped off all kinds of food—casseroles, sandwiches, trays of fresh fruit and vegetables. They brought cut flower arrangements, pretty potted plants, and bulbs and seeds for the garden. It was thoughtful. Kind.

The bulbs nearly cost me my sanity. They sat in the garage, applying such pressure to my already overcrowded mind.

Don't they know I'm not the gardener? How could they not know it was Kevin who loved to make things grow? I put the bulbs on top of the garbage can more than once, but each time I saw them, I thought, *Kevin would hate that.*

Dirt had not made its way beneath my fingernails since kindergarten, when I planted sunflower seeds in a tiny Styrofoam cup for Mother's day.

How was I supposed to plant the bulbs? Where?

One warm Saturday, I asked the kids to pick up soil with fertilizer in it. They brought four fifty-pound sacks. I planted a few flowers around the mailbox.

Okay, that wasn't so bad, I thought. Then I sprinkled a few seeds around the front walk. That was easy, too, so I tossed handfuls of seeds.

The bulbs were not easy. They wore skins like onions that shed. Was I supposed to peel them off or not? I did. Which side was supposed to be planted facing up? Was it the pointy side or the flat side with the fringy hair? *Hair,* I thought. Hair has roots and roots go down.

Calling to Katie, I asked her to dump one whole sack of the soil and fertilizer in the backyard. It didn't matter where, so she slit open the bag and emptied it right where she opened it.

As the dark fell on my gardening attempt, I started crying, hard. I was hungry, sweaty, dirty, and frustrated. I felt so stupid.

Why am I out here? I shouldn't be doing this! Kevin was the one who loved gardening. He should be here. Where is he? How did this happen?

Tears and snot ran down my face, dripping into the new garden I'd made, which was only a pile of mud and mucus.

In a few weeks, though, the bulbs shot out of the ground with new life, wholly redeemed.

My physical stress symptoms erupted after Kevin died. My foot hurt. When I finally had time to get it checked out, a broken bone showed up on the x-ray. It was a bone I'd fractured once before. All that squatting on my legs next to Kevin's recliner had put so much stress on it that the weakened bone fractured again. I hadn't even noticed. Every time I drove by the hospital, heart palpitations flared in my chest. Strange rashes appeared on my skin. My joints hurt. These outward signs were manifestations of the grief, the horrible confusion, the fear, the depthless pain. The severity of my physical symptoms of grief shocked me.

I failed him. The whole system failed him. I'm just so grateful we had what we had for as long as we did. I'm not ready to let it go. What happened? I still don't understand it. I feel so broken. So wounded. I long for things to be the way they were and miss you more than I could ever imagine. I long for those normal days. I hate this life now. Unprotected. Unsupported. Alone.

When I talked to the kids, their grief was almost too much to bear, and I questioned my mothering constantly. Only a little while ago, they'd had a father they got along with, went to games with, talked with. Then no father. Worse still, a dead father.

Now they're stuck with me. Maybe they think I didn't cry enough. Maybe I was too strong, too tough, ice cold. That's what I had to be. There were only so many compartments, so many drawers in my mind to close things into so I could save them for later and carry on doing what I had to do.

There were no rules for the grief. No milestones. It was the Soggy Year. The Year of Constant Sobbing. The Year of Uneven Ground. The Year No Rules Applied. The Year I Wished to Flush.

When is the grief enough? I wondered. A truly good man was gone. One of the good guys. How was I supposed to show my sadness? Why did I care who saw it? When was it enough?

I thought I knew about crying. But the crying I did then was unbelievable. During Kevin's illness, I sobbed internally, my shoulders aching. I couldn't let anyone see me cry. After he died, the grief overcame me. I cried in my sleep and woke up to a wet pillow. I didn't know what to do. I tried to go for walks, but putting one leg out of bed was too much. I just couldn't do it. Most mornings, my youngest daughter left for school by herself while I stayed in bed. I didn't eat, didn't drink, didn't sleep. I stayed in my pajamas and only managed to get up and moving moments before Christine walked in the door from school. Once she was home, I couldn't wait to go back to bed. I never felt refreshed or completely awake.

Early and deep grief behaviors have characteristics like mental illness. *Bipolar Disorder.* I laughed hysterically one minute and bawled the next. *Schizophrenia.* I swear I heard the garage door open at the same time Kevin normally returned home from work. Other times I heard his voice, and once I thought I saw him out of the corner of my eye. *Catatonia.* I could not get out of bed. I didn't care to, and my body wouldn't allow it. *Sleep Disturbances.* Deep sleep was impossible.

Crying in my sleep was the reality, and I had multiple lucid dreams in which I felt fully awake.

The truth is I thought I was losing my mind. During that dark time, I thought I would be better off dead. I saw the butcher knife in the kitchen and thought how I could put it to such good use.

Where are you?! Why am I here and you're not? Just tell me one more thing—tell me one more of your philosophies about math or science. They made so much sense when you said them. Nothing makes sense now. What am I supposed to do?

I was embarrassed.

How could this have happened in your house?

I felt under constant scrutiny. Attention at work and attention when I picked Christine up from school. I couldn't just be a normal person. In my mind, I couldn't run to the grocery store without makeup on. I thought I had to put on a good front because everybody was constantly checking on me and patting me on the shoulder. "How are you doing today?" I had to get dressed up so people wouldn't think I was doing poorly.

On paper, Kevin should have made it. He had a gold-plated insurance card, a nurse practitioner for a wife. He had every benefit you can imagine, and his death made me feel like a failure in every way.

Kevin never thought he was going to die. He truly believed he was in that one percent of people who make it two years. Kevin often told me his philosophy of life: "No means yes and yes means yes," he'd say. And for him, it was true. He could talk anybody into anything. But that outlook betrayed him with the cancer treatment.

If you knew it was just going to be a couple months of time you had left, would you have spent it the way you did? I know what you'd say. "What were we thinking? We should have just been together."

DEATH ENVY

Nobody told me what happens after your spouse dies. Many times, I thought I'd be better off dead. I ruminated about the benefits of death. I wouldn't have to vacuum or run to the grocery store. I wouldn't have to take a shower, which seemed like such a huge task at the time. I learned later that these thoughts are normal for the widowed spouse.

Clinicians get worried when someone starts planning to die. If I'd purchased a gun or bought poison, I'd be put in a different category of concern. But death envy happens to many of us. If we learn how normal it is, then talking can take the sting out of the experience.

I remember thinking, *I could die now if I wanted to, but there is a good movie on tonight*. Distracting myself helped me choose life every day instead of giving up.

THERAPY

After Kevin died, people asked if I had signed my children up for grief counseling. The answer was no. They didn't want therapy, and I didn't push it. My own experience with counseling didn't offer me the instant fix I wanted, so we didn't turn to counselors for help. Instead, we relied on each other, our family, and our friends.

Researchers Joseph M. Currier, Robert A. Neimeyer, and Jeffrey S. Berman revealed something surprising in their study "The Effectiveness of Psychotherapeutic Interventions for Bereaved Persons: A Comprehensive Quantitative Review" (*Psychological Bulletin*, 2008). Normally, we would expect that people who receive counseling get better and that people who don't receive counseling get worse. Instead, the researchers found that everyone gets better.

People with acute grief symptoms that lasted longer than six months did find counseling helpful, though.

To me, this research confirms what I found to be true. I couldn't follow a prescribed method of healing. I had to stitch together my own tapestry of resources.

chapter fourteen

alone

I dealt with the busywork. Lawyers, accountants, financial advisors, workmen. After I visited the cancer center one last time, I sent the staff a pretty arrangement of cut fruit. I wished them well and thanked them for keeping Kevin's chart so well organized.

I felt incapable of the tasks required to keep our lives running. The house was comfortable and pretty, yet the demands of maintaining it sucked the life out of me. The children needed me constantly. I wondered in my depression and overwhelming loss: Would I have given birth to them if I'd known they'd have to experience the loss of their father?

The financial people swooped in like vultures. After a lifetime of ignoring money and letting Kevin handle it, I was suddenly responsible for the cash that came at too terrible a price. Financial advisors liken widows to lottery winners and assume they know nothing about money. In my case, this was true. I felt stupid and ill-equipped. Kevin's life insurance company sent a team of three people to talk to me. I don't know what made me take my father with me, but I'm glad I did. They wanted to sell their products right away, but I wasn't prepared for that kind of conversation.

At the same time, I couldn't remember how to order checks. Even though the old me had done it a million times, the new me couldn't remember how. I showed up one day at a printer in town asking them to print me up some more checks. When they sent me away saying they couldn't do it, I felt so stupid but it was all I could think to do.

While I struggled, I thanked Kevin often for carefully tending our estate plans, insurance, and finances.

I set short-term goals: returning to work, listening to the kids, getting them ready for school. I kept forgetting things—sentences I was about to say or papers I'd set down. I wanted to change telephone service providers. After waiting fourteen minutes, some faceless, bland young woman named Amanda said she would like to speak with Kevin, since the account was in his name. I told her Kevin died. She put me on hold. When she returned several minutes later, she told me that I had to send a death certificate and a copy of my ID before they could change the name to mine.

My lawyers had advised me to not give out copies of the death certificate, since it could lead to identity theft.

"I'm not sending you the death certificate," I said. "I'll cancel my account and reapply for a new one on my own."

"Oh, no," the young woman said. "You can't do that either since you're not named on the bill."

I felt my pulse rise and asked for her supervisor. A mind-numbing thirty-nine minutes later, the supervisor agreed that I couldn't make any changes to my account without the two documents.

"It's just like switching college roommates," he said. "It's not a big deal." It was against their policy, he went on, because I could be a malicious caller who wanted to mess up someone else's cable service.

My choices were to submit the documents my lawyers had said to keep carefully guarded or let the bill go to collections. I even went to their office and physically showed them the documents, but they still wouldn't close the account. As far as I know, it's still open.

I sought counseling for $125 an hour. The 125 bucks would have done more good if I'd gone shopping. Since I felt so nuts, I wanted to make sure I was normal. The therapist listened. Back then I was fixated on the medical events: *How did this happen?*

I thought I would walk out of the session and say, "I'm so much better! Check that one off the list." What could somebody say to make it better?

The counselor didn't do anything wrong, he just listened, but it wasn't what I was looking for. I wanted him to bless me and say, "Good job! Now go back to work."

I dreaded returning to my job. I started slowly, working for a few hours a week after seven weeks off. It was hard. I didn't have anything to offer my patients. I didn't want to talk and couldn't listen. Some days I could feel empathy for them, some days I couldn't. Internally I cycled through disbelief, sorrow, and rage. Work was a chore. Being at home was a chore. I lived in a house full of memories and regret. No matter how many fleece jackets I wore, I couldn't shake the chill I felt.

I don't know how to be a widow. It feels like it'll pass. It feels like any minute now, I'll hear the garage door open and he'll walk in.

I desperately missed the everydayness of my old life. Thursdays were always pizza nights at our house. Those normal, predictable routines added up to a good life, and I craved them.

No one could validate my stories anymore. My daughter told a friend about something she thought Kevin had done, but in reality it had been me. Kevin wasn't there to validate my memory, my reality.

The painter saved my life. He doesn't know that, but he did. By the time Kevin was sick, we'd had the house for years and had talked about how it needed a new coat of paint to cover the dinged up walls. I knew I didn't want a crew of painters around, so a friend introduced me to Paul. He painted my home with such careful attention.

We talked a little bit every day. He kept the pets company. His gentle presence reduced the dread I felt every day when I returned. The house had become an empty shell, a prison. As soon as the kids walked in from school or I got home from work, he politely left.

We had huge, pitched walls, but he never complained or asked for help. Whenever I came home, everything was packed up and returned to where it belonged. He was the extra pair of hands I didn't know I needed.

Paul seemed to love the house. He transformed it into a different place with every stroke of the brush. He made me see color and light. When choosing paint, he encouraged me to choose color over vanilla blandness and sameness. I translated that philosophy to my own life. Perhaps it was time to choose something other than desperate longing. The longing for a life that was over, that was so completely, totally gone that it could never be resuscitated.

Paul, the therapist, philosopher, and painter, was very practical and matter-of-fact. Nothing stopped him. He easily moved my heavy furniture where it had to go like it was no big deal. And he set an example for me. He just kept showing up, doing the job every day. And as he transformed my home, I felt something shift in my heart. Maybe I would be okay.

I had a dream. In our early life together, we spent a lot of time in airports. Kevin and I shared huge, weeping "I love you, I'll miss you" moments with big, long kisses. The welcome home scenes were equally dramatic. Those times were fabulous and romantic.

In my dream, I ran through an airport, frantically looking for Kevin. So many people walked by. I struggled, fighting through the wrong way in a massive crowd. Finally, I saw him walking toward me in his navy blue Dockers and a light-colored polo shirt. His eyes stared straight ahead. He was happy. He had no baggage. It was the man I knew and loved every day. The only difference was that he wasn't looking for me.

Kevin had wanted to live until July so that he could attend his niece's wedding. I put the urn filled with his cremains in the backseat of my car. "Cremains" is the word they use for the remains of the body left after cremation. When I brought the urn home, I put it in the closet beneath Kevin's clothes. Chip, the cat that screamed the moment Kevin died, found it and regularly sat on top of it.

Every time I looked in that closet, Kevin's stuff weighed heavily on me. I had to deal with his belongings.

What do I keep? What do I throw away?

For a while, I kept everything because I didn't want to touch it. Since chemo leaks through your pores, I was afraid that Kevin had left chemo drugs on whatever he touched. But I finally cleaned everything out. It had become unbearable to look at the belongings we shared together. He had seventy-six polo shirts in his closet that he hadn't worn since he got sick. I bagged them all up and paid a kid to deliver them to Goodwill. The sappy love letters we wrote to each other, all tied up in a pretty ribbon, were goners. Kevin saved every paycheck he ever received. I threw them all away. I just couldn't bear it.

Medicines, creams, and ointments—all the paraphernalia of sickness—cluttered the bathroom. I chucked it all. I even sold both our cars and bought a new one.

I'd heard that some widowed women would wear their ring on the other hand or wear it on a chain around their neck or have it melted down and made into something else. I didn't want to take my wedding ring off, but since I'd lost so much weight, it fell off one day while I washed dishes.

The day it came off, I didn't slip it back on. Instead, I put it in my dresser drawer. I found that I missed the weight of the ring. On really bad days—our anniversary, Kevin's birthday, or days when the loss was heavy on my heart—I grabbed the ring and slept with it on overnight. I always took it off in the morning so the girls wouldn't see it.

After six months, my life was unrecognizable. Longtime friends all but disappeared, the telephone stopped ringing, and the couple friends we saw bimonthly were history.

I was alone. No husband. Kids launching. No one was coming to my rescue. There were times in my married life that I wanted to be alone. Not anymore. Smug couples walked by me holding hands, and envy overwhelmed me.

Social Security says I'm free to remarry. Do they have somebody in mind?

I was released from my marriage. I liked being married. I liked my husband, and I liked our partnership. I liked it better in the early years, when there was less stress and fewer demands on our time, but we had retirement to think of and could put our relationship on hold because we had time. We looked forward to the mellow years to come and renegotiating our contract with each other.

If we had only known . . . I don't think we would have done much differently, do you? Am I wrong? Did you hate your life? I don't think you did. You had it pretty good, I think. So did I. That's the problem. I want my old life back.

I tried to remember when we became estranged, when we became short with one another and testy and tired. When we lost compassion and even treated each other with contempt. I tried to figure that out, but there was no one to balance out my memories. Kevin couldn't tell his side of the story.

A long list of "shoulds" assailed me. I shouldn't have nagged so much. I should have given him more credit. I should have insisted on certain things. I should have renegotiated my marriage. Kevin should still be alive.

I desperately searched for resources that would help me. I read books about the "gift" of dying. Gift? I couldn't see how it was a gift. Books that tried to reassure me that Kevin was "in a better place" made me want to puke.

In my search to normalize my feelings, I went to a meeting of a widow / widowers support group. It was so awful. I was younger than everyone by at least two decades, and my loss was the most recent. It felt like a singles mixer, and I never went back. There was a young widow / widowers support group about forty minutes away, but whenever I found the courage to call for dates, they said it was canceled due to lack of participants. However, if I learned that someone I met had lost a spouse, I talked to them one-on-one. It helped far more than the books.

That year I went to Barnes and Noble to get Katie her Halloween card, just like every year. I could barely look at the colorful cards. "From our family to yours." "Wish you were here."

I did. Wish he was here. Would I appreciate him? Would I miss him and run to the door every night he came home? It still felt as if he had gone on a very long trip.

I wish you were here.

There was so much I couldn't do, but my body remembered how to walk. Sometimes I walked for four hours. I numbered my steps or just counted up to one hundred and started again. I had this crushing feeling of being alone. Stranded. Nothing to do, and all day to do it.

I didn't recognize myself. Not only was I down a strong domestic partner, I wasn't married anymore. I had to check the "widow" box when I filled out forms. Instead of engaging in life, my movement was robotic. I said the right things, smiled in the right places, but numbness enveloped me.

Don't look at me. Don't touch me. Some days, I feel like I could shatter.

When I went out, I saw people who knew us. I wondered what they thought. Was I supposed to be sitting home alone, wrapped in my grief? There were no rules to widowhood. No guidelines to check off, month after month, to assess my progress.

I planned ahead for events like my work holiday party and always found someone to sit next to me. Kevin used to pull my chair out for me. One of us would make sure we had a place to sit, and then he'd go to the bar for our cocktails. In the tradition of long-married couples, our routines in social situations were so familiar to me. That married part of us was always in gear.

When he was gone, I had to learn how to fill his role, too. I had to learn how to sign leases, buy and sell houses, deal with bankers, put my own luggage in the overhead bins on the airplane.

For a while, I continued to do what I thought Kevin would want me to do. As the year anniversary of Kevin's death approached, new thoughts bloomed.

Stop it. His turn is over. How long will you keep your life in suspended animation?

In another dream, I heard Kevin's voice in my mind: "Get back in the game!"

GRIEF

What does your grief look like? Do you know what is normal for someone grieving the death of a loved one? I didn't. And after I researched both consumer and clinical books on grief, I still didn't. The medical community has made an illness out of grief, but grieving is completely normal. Everyone accepts that the loss is forever, so it's natural to feel the loss in some form for your entire life. The accepted medical definition of grief says it's supposed to last about a year. If you have severe grief symptoms, such as depression, despair, anxiety, yearning, intrusive thoughts, and shock, that last too long—more than a year—you are classified as someone with complicated grief.

The most well known information on grief is based on Elisabeth Kübler-Ross's five stages of grief, but according to new studies, those stages aren't necessarily helpful for everyone. They were originally meant for a person facing their own death, not the death of someone else.

There are other general things that people go through. You really start grieving on the day of diagnosis. There are people who can do their grief work while their loved one is dying and they come out of the experience feeling healthy. If that happens to you, it's not something to feel badly about.

Some people experience intense grief. You believe you're thinking normally, but you may not be. Do the best you can. Take care of yourself without doing something you'll regret later. Some surviving spouses might think it's an affirmation of life to jump out of an airplane or do other wacky stuff. Or remarry too soon. Starting to date and travel were ways to distract myself around the first anniversary of my husband's death, and those activities helped me come back to life.

If you think you're suffering from acute grief, don't feel ashamed or embarrassed to seek out help. Please, let yourself off the hook. You're doing the best you can.

OVER

In an episode of the famous television show Sex in the City, the main character, Carrie Bradshaw, has just broken up with her boyfriend Big (again). She narrates, "We're so over, we need a new word for over." Even now, five years after Kevin died, "over" is the best word I can use to describe the experience. It's over.

chapter fifteen
waking up

Hey Mom,

I just want you to know I'm thinking about you lots. I hope you're having a wonderful time and getting all that you need from this trip. I hope when you come back, you feel unbelievably refreshed and maybe even ready to move on with your life.

We know you won't forget your husband, but you don't need to suffer anymore for it. You did all that you could. He had the best possible end-of-life care anyone has ever had. Nothing you did could have changed it. He never stood a chance against that awful cancer. It's time for you to stop regretting the things you two didn't do and start celebrating the things you did.

He loved you an unbelievable amount. Told everyone you were his angel.

Stop punishing yourself. Stop regretting the time that wasn't perfect. I do remember the wonderful couple you were, all the way to the end.

Love, Katie

About nine months into widowhood, I started thinking about how to spend the anniversary of Kevin's death. It was December, and I'd already lived through the anniversary of his diagnosis and the holidays without him. I knew I could stay and be with the girls, but a thought crept into my mind that I couldn't shake.

I don't have to stay here.

For several months I had researched trips, looking at excursions that included transportation so I wouldn't have to drive. I wanted something that felt safe so I wouldn't worry about being alone. Finally, I found the perfect trip.

Before booking my spot, I talked with my daughters and told them my plan. They were older now, seventeen and twenty-one, and Katie, my oldest, had married her boyfriend. They both said they'd be fine spending the time together without me, and I trusted they spoke the truth. It was time I honored Kevin in my own way. I wanted to be the wife again and take private time for the grief. I didn't need to be at the house where he'd died.

I booked myself a flight to New Orleans and took a leisurely ride back on a luxury train. The train traveled at night, and during the day, the tour guides escorted us around the cities on our stops. I always ditched the escort to explore on my own. I walked through each town for six hours at a time, exploring cities along the way including Savannah, Georgia, and Washington, D.C.

The travel was so therapeutic for me. It felt wonderful to be alone and not have to talk to people if I didn't want to. For the first time since the diagnosis, I didn't feel scrutinized by well-meaning neighbors or colleagues. I didn't have to pretend I was fine. I could give in to my grief a little bit. I could be alone with how I felt.

As the miles passed beneath my feet and rolled under the cars of the train, I started to wake up. I noticed things I hadn't noticed in a long time—flowers, people, new sights. I made myself do one new thing every single day, even though the sadness was still my companion. I experienced moments of longing so strong that I felt the ache in my body.

How could you be gone? I can't talk to you about how I feel about you being gone. That's not right. We talked about every little thing.

The cherry blossoms were in bloom when we arrived in Washington, D.C. I reserved a hotel room near the train station and set out on a gorgeous day for another long walk. I noticed a sign for the Allen Chapel African Methodist Episcopal Church. People swarmed the building. I went to see what was happening and found two elderly gentlemen sitting near the door to the church.

"We're getting ready for a fish fry supper," one of the men explained.

"Do you need any help?" I asked.

"No, but you can come back when we're serving," the other said.

"I will," I said.

"You're not coming back." They both ribbed me, taking bets about whether or not I'd return for the food, as though we'd known each other our entire lives.

Walking on, I passed a kite-flying festival and watched the erratic dance of colorful fabrics buoyed by the wind. Later I made my way to the Smithsonian, where there was a nursing history exhibit. I didn't go in. I just walked and walked, forgetting lunch, forgetting everything but the hypnotic rhythm of my steps.

On the way back to my hotel, I stopped by the Allen Chapel. The entire congregation welcomed me and seated me at a table with other single people. I paid ten dollars for the best food I'd ever had. It was the first time I tasted a Hush Puppy.

In our early days together, Kevin, our girls, and I used to go to church suppers. Sitting there, the only white woman in a black congregation filled with loving people, I finally felt refreshed.

I'm feeling better, I realized. And that was okay. I gave myself permission to start feeling better. Whenever I noticed the clock hit 11:11, I asked Kevin a question, or simply thanked him. As I returned from my trip, instead of wondering what Kevin would have done, I started asking myself, "Well, what are *you* going to do?"

The day I came back from the train trip, I returned from my own journey through shock, grief, and guilt. I was ready to make some changes. After that trip, my mind opened up. I realized that I was independent. I didn't have to do the same things I'd always done.

I'd taken on the role of the widow, but I started feeling like I didn't have to anymore. When Kevin died, I put my life on hold for a year and did nothing but continue breathing. The train trip made me appreciate being outside again, eating delicious food again.

There was a waiter on the train who knew I liked desserts, and when I returned to my cabin, there would be an extra dessert waiting for me. In his own way, he spoiled me—and I needed a little spoiling.

I booked massages and treated myself to flowers. Kevin never liked garlic or salmon, and I started eating salmon all the time. It was a strain to figure out what to eat because there were so many choices, and I didn't want to say no to myself anymore. Sometimes I purchased salmon *and* steak if I couldn't decide.

We'd been an active couple before, but I'd stopped going out. So on Fridays I made myself pick a movie I wanted to see. I'd go to the 4:00 p.m. matinee and sit in the dark with a root beer and a bag of popcorn. At first, I watched the other people who were by themselves. They looked fine, while I felt so uncomfortable being out alone. Over time, I stopped feeling self-conscious. I went out to dinner, saw plays, and soaked in the energy of the crowd. Going out alone turned out to be a fun experience that I continue to do today.

In a newsletter from a local widow / widowers support group, I read, "Allow yourself the privilege of limping until your wounds have healed and you can learn to run again."

I wish someone had said this to me.

At the end of that first year, I thought life would regain some semblance of normalcy. It didn't. The work was just different. I focused on redefining myself, but I had to acknowledge each small step I took toward recovery.

I just got the mail and didn't have to rest before I opened it.
I felt like baking a loaf of bread and actually did it.
I remembered to pay the bills on time.

I woke up one day and found I wasn't crying. I was able to have a second cup of coffee. I could think about carnations with a smile. When we were young and broke and in love, Kevin would bring me carnations every week because they were all he could afford. Even when he could send me fancier flowers, he always had carnations wrapped up and sent to where I worked.

Instead of rehashing the painful parts of Kevin's journey through cancer, or the tough times in our marriage, or the words I regretted, I allowed myself to open up to the wonderful memories. It was okay to let those warm feelings come over me. They weren't going to kill me or make me sadder.

About three months after that wonderful trip, I moved out of Kevin's dream house. I didn't want to spend my time doing yard work.

And even though I tried hard to pretend I liked gardening—because I thought every widow was a good gardener—I hated it. The house was too big. I'd scoured the MLS for a new place to live, but a friend found a small house right on the water that seemed to fit. The house was tiny, the lot small. It was perfect, so I moved in June. And it was good. Another step. Another stretch as I woke.

I decided to go back to school to study palliative care and hospice work. I dug into cancer data, wanting to understand how Kevin's death had happened even though he'd been to one of the highest rated cancer centers in the world.

I felt more energy than I had in a long time. After Kevin's death, I realized my own time was ticking away, so I signed up for more classes. I traveled. I pushed myself out of my comfort zone. I did more things away from my children, since they had graduated from college and high school and built their own lives. Time did its work. I was coming into my own.

My friends told me later there was some talk that I wouldn't be on the market for long—bets were that I'd be married in a year or less. I found it both offensive and flattering. Did my friends think I couldn't handle life alone? At the same time, I was secretly pleased that they saw me as fit material for dating. I said yes to some safe dates with friends of friends. Kevin had suggested a few men he thought I should date, and I did—except for the one who was married. I had a wonderful time with some very nice guys, but I couldn't imagine ever marrying again. I couldn't bear the thought of seeing someone else through an illness.

That first year, I held everything the same: the traditions, the routines. I wanted everything to be the same in the face of such shattering change. I could have chosen to stay the same forever.

But I realized, during that vacation on the first anniversary of Kevin's death, that I couldn't help but change.

After I learned more about cancer and end-of-life issues at school, I wished I could go back to the moment Kevin was diagnosed. I would have demanded we talk about the benefits *and* burdens of treatment. But the truth is we didn't know anything at the time. All we had was our desperate desire for him to live. If Kevin had known he would die so quickly after the traumatic chemotherapy and radiation, it might have broken him in some way worse than it did. At the end of the day, we made the best choices we could make at the time.

I continue to make the best choices I can make right now, in this moment, in this new life without my husband. And even though he's not with me, I still check in with him from time to time. After Kevin died, the operations manager at GE retired Kevin's old office telephone number to honor him. I call it still. The voice mail doesn't pick up. It just rings and rings, but I know Kevin's out there somewhere. On a trip. Having the time of his life.

And me? Aren't you proud, honey? I'm back in the game.

THE FIVE TASKS OF LIFE COMPLETION

I'm sorry.
I forgive you.
Do you forgive me?
I love you.
Good-bye.

chapter sixteen
just five more minutes

Helping people with their advance directives or health care directives is a big part of what palliative care clinicians do. Once a patient is diagnosed with a life-limiting illness, I sit down and talk to them about what life-saving measures they want or don't want in the event that they can't speak for themselves. An advance directive, also called a living will, is a written tool that guides health care decisions if you're incapable of making them yourself. It's important to write up your own advance directives right now, whether you're sick or not, young or old.

Each state has its own laws and offers forms that guide you through the process, with specific questions about:

- Medical care treatments
- Religious and spiritual beliefs
- Feelings about quality and length of life
- Preferences for care when dying

- Wishes about donating organs, tissues, or other body parts
- Importance of pain control
- Wishes for the use of life-prolonging treatment under a variety of circumstances

If you've filled out an advance directive but moved to another state, or if you spend a lot of time in a different state, you need to make sure you have everything needed for the states where you live or work.

I have so many patients who say, "I want a good quality of life. You can deep-freeze me until you find a cure for my disease." The truth is we don't have that kind of technology right now. You need to understand what each decision really means. Having an advance directive eases the burden on your family, so please don't put it off. You can find the documents you need with a simple online search.

Patients often write up advance directives without knowing what they're signing up for. A ventilator (vent), for instance, was never meant to be a long-term way to keep the body alive. It is supposed to be a bridge until the patient can breathe on his or her own. The vent is invasive and the machine is loud. For short-term care, it can be the perfect solution. If someone is in a car or skiing accident, they might go on a vent until the lung bruising goes away.

It's the same with dialysis. It was designed for end-stage kidney shutdown. It was never meant to be life sustaining. After kidney failure, dialysis filters the toxins out, but it takes the good stuff too, including blood pressure medications and antidepressants. People have to be hooked to the dialysis machine for an average of six hours. They will feel better the next day, but towards the end they'll start feeling worse again. By the third day, they have to go back for more.

Dialysis for a short amount of time does make sense. And you can time limit the usage in your advance directive.

If you're on a ventilator because you have cancer or have suffered a trauma, it makes sense for a few days. But the cancer is still growing. Your family needs to know when to stop the vent, and the time for these discussions is not five minutes before you have to be intubated.

You also need to decide whether or not to have cardiopulmonary resuscitation (CPR). You've probably seen hundreds of television shows where the heart stops. There's a flurry of activity. The doctor administers CPR and the patient wakes up and smiles. That only happens seventeen to twenty-two percent of the time. CPR works best in a young, healthy person for accidents involving electric current, near-drowning, or vehicles.

In a disease like cancer, where the patient is already dying from another process, CPR only works about five percent of the time and makes no sense in cases like this. It puts a lot of stress on the body. The patient will have their chest compressed, and if the cancer is in the late stages or in the bones, the patient's ribs can crack and break. It is horrifically traumatic to both the patient *and* the person giving the CPR. When a patient is already in the late stages of cancer and all the medications in the world wouldn't help, CPR is wildly inappropriate.

Sometimes a person will come back to life after CPR and be placed on the ventilator, too. Once on a ventilator, you're not capable of participating in your medical decisions anymore because you can't talk. So someone else will make the decision when or if to remove that tube.

You don't need a lawyer to fill out an advance directive, but the documents do need to be notarized. All hospitals have a social worker who will notarize it for free. If you're brought to the hospital, the admitting clerk must ask for your advance directive. Please, don't tell them it's at your lawyer's office. Always have a copy in your personal papers or even in your wallet. Have your physician put a copy in your medical file. Give a copy to the person you've selected to be your voice. That person, called your health care agent, or proxy, has durable power of attorney and can be anybody you wish, such as a family member or friend. And you should designate alternate health care agents in case the first one is unable to help. The proxy has the legal right to make health care decisions for you within the limits you've spelled out in your advance directives.

In some states, the power of attorney is part of the advance health care directive documents. In other states, you have to file a separate document. This type of power of attorney does not include the legal right to handle your financial affairs. (That is the executor of your estate, and that requires different documents.) You might pick the same person to do both, but you don't have to.

It's important to know that power of attorney is not legally activated until your physician assesses your condition to see if you can participate in medical decision-making. A judge or lawyer decides if you're capable of making financial decisions.

If you're awake, in order to make your own medical decisions, you need to know the date, where you are, the nature of your injury or illness, and the risks and benefits of expected treatment.

When you choose someone to be your voice, it's important to go over your wishes with him or her. If they can't honor your wishes, you'll have to choose someone else. I've seen this happen numerous times. For instance, someone's religious beliefs change and they can't follow through with your instructions. Once you can't speak for yourself, the wishes of whoever is speaking for you will be honored.

It's smart to update your directives every couple of years and check in with the people you've designated as your health care agents, including all the alternates. The fact is we call the people in the order that you've listed them. Whoever we reach first gets the job.

planning for your funeral

I always advise people to take ten minutes out of your busy schedule to review your death plans. Do not leave these matters to your surviving spouse or family members. Pour a glass of wine if you like and briefly go over the list of questions below.

Do you want to be buried or cremated?

If you want to be buried, do you have a cemetery in mind?

Do you want a monument? What do you want it to say?

Do you want a funeral?

If yes, what kind of music do you want? Where do you want it to be held? Do you have favorite readings or stories you want read? Who will write and read your eulogy?

Do you want to have an open casket?

If you don't want a funeral, how do you want people to be able to say goodbye to you?

Do you want a wake?

What do you want to wear to your funeral?

How will your loved ones pay for the casket, funeral, burial, or cremation?

Do you want to donate your organs for medical purposes or your body for scientific research? Medical and scientific donations require you to pay the funeral home to prepare the body and transport it to wherever you're donating to.

Do you have life insurance that will cover all your spouse's needs?

WIDOW

There are very few resources that tell you anything about becoming a widow. Every one of us has to carve out what it looks like for us. I remember hearing this advice a lot: Don't make any decisions for a year. That didn't work for me. I had to make decisions. I couldn't help it. Everything had already changed.

I think widows need the permission to do whatever they need to do. So please, allow me. *I give you permission to do what you need to do to get well.*

You can steep in death, in the unfairness, the disruption, the sadness of it, or you can see it for the release it may represent. You don't get a vote in when somebody else dies. You may object vehemently. But you didn't die. There are no rules here, but eventually you must release the life you had before and move forward to create a new one.

about the author

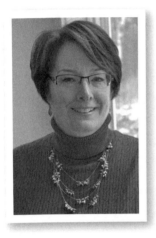

Lynn Kelly Devlin is a nationally board certified Hospice and Palliative Care nurse practitioner who lives and works in New Hampshire. She often speaks to health care professionals, corporate audiences, students, and small groups about end-of-life issues. www.lynndevlin.com

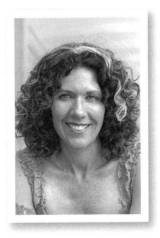

Jacquelyn B. Fletcher is an award-winning author. Her books include *Climbing the Mountain: Stories of Hope and Healing after Stroke and Brain Injury* (Fairview Press) and *A Career Girl's Guide to Becoming a Stepmom* (HarperCollins). www.jacquelynfletcher.com